Harm Reduction Treatment for Substance Use

About the Authors

Susan E. Collins, PhD, (she/her) is a licensed clinical psychologist, faculty at the University of Washington School of Medicine and Washington State University, co-director of the Harm Reduction Research and Treatment (HaRRT) Center, and co-founder of the social purpose corporation, HaRT3S. Dr. Collins has been involved in substance use research, assessment, and treatment for over 25 years and has disseminated this work in over seven dozen book chapters, abstracts, and peer-reviewed articles. Dr. Collins also brings her own lived experience as a person in recovery from addictive behaviors and as a woman embedded in families with the intergenerational experience of addictive behaviors, substance use disorder, and substance-related harm.

Seema L. Clifasefi, PhD, is a licensed clinical social worker, an associate professor and co-director of the Harm Reduction Research and Treatment (HaRRT) Center at the University of Washington – Harborview Medical Center, and co-founder of the social purpose corporation HaRT3S. Her research lies at the intersection of substance use, mental health, criminal justice, and housing policy. For the past nearly two decades she has been part of several collaborative academic/community-based research partnerships focused on the development and evaluation of individual and community-level harm reduction programs and interventions designed for and with people who have lived experience of homelessness and substance use problems.

Advances in Psychotherapy – Evidence-Based Practice

Series Editor
Danny Wedding, PhD, MPH, Professor Emeritus, University of Missouri–Saint Louis, MO

Associate Editors
Jonathan S. Comer, PhD, Professor of Psychology and Psychiatry, Director of Mental Health Interventions and Technology (MINT) Program, Center for Children and Families, Florida International University, Miami, FL

J. Kim Penberthy, PhD, ABPP, Professor of Psychiatry & Neurobehavioral Sciences, University of Virginia, Charlottesville, VA

Kenneth E. Freedland, PhD, Professor of Psychiatry and Psychology, Washington University School of Medicine, St. Louis, MO

Linda C. Sobell, PhD, ABPP, Professor, Center for Psychological Studies, Nova Southeastern University, Ft. Lauderdale, FL

The basic objective of this series is to provide therapists with practical, evidence-based treatment guidance for the most common disorders seen in clinical practice – and to do so in a reader-friendly manner. Each book in the series is both a compact "how-to" reference on a particular disorder for use by professional clinicians in their daily work and an ideal educational resource for students as well as for practice-oriented continuing education.

The most important feature of the books is that they are practical and easy to use: All are structured similarly and all provide a compact and easy-to-follow guide to all aspects that are relevant in real-life practice. Tables, boxed clinical "pearls," marginal notes, and summary boxes assist orientation, while checklists provide tools for use in daily practice.

Continuing Education Credits

Psychologists and other healthcare providers may earn five continuing education credits for reading the books in the *Advances in Psychotherapy* series and taking a multiple-choice exam. This continuing education program is a partnership of Hogrefe Publishing and the National Register of Health Service Psychologists. Details are available at https://www.hogrefe.com/us/cenatreg

The National Register of Health Service Psychologists is approved by the American Psychological Association to sponsor continuing education for psychologists. The National Register maintains responsibility for this program and its content.

Advances in Psychotherapy – Evidence-Based Practice, Volume 49

Harm Reduction Treatment for Substance Use

Susan E. Collins
HaRRT Center, Department of Psychiatry and Behavioral Sciences, University of Washington, School of Medicine, Seattle, WA
Department of Psychology, Washington State University, Pullman, WA

Seema L. Clifasefi
HaRRT Center, Department of Psychiatry and Behavioral Sciences, University of Washington, School of Medicine, Seattle, WA

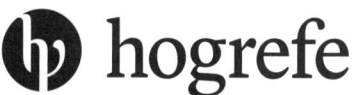

Library of Congress of Congress Cataloging in Publication information for the print version of this book is available via the Library of Congress Marc Database under the Library of Congress Control Number 2023933421

Library and Archives Canada Cataloguing in Publication

Title: Harm reduction treatment for substance use / Susan E. Collins (HaRRT Center, Department of Psychiatry and Behavioral Sciences, University of Washington, School of Medicine, Seattle, WA, Department of Psychology, Washington State University, Pullman, WA), Seema L. Clifasefi (HaRRT Center, Department of Psychiatry and Behavioral Sciences, University of Washington, School of Medicine, Seattle, WA).

Names: Collins, Susan E., author. | Clifasefi, Seema L., author.

Series: Advances in psychotherapy--evidence-based practice ; v. 49.

Description: Series statement: Advances in psychotherapy--evidence-based practice ; volume 49 | Includes bibliographical references.

Identifiers: Canadiana (print) 20230194028 | Canadiana (ebook) 20230194087 | ISBN 9780889375079 (softcover) | ISBN 9781613345078 (EPUB) | ISBN 9781616765071 (PDF)

Subjects: LCSH: Substance abuse—Treatment. | LCSH: Substance abuse—Social aspects. | LCSH: Harm reduction. | LCSH: Psychotherapy.

Classification: LCC RC564 .C65 2023 | DDC 616.86/06—dc23

© 2023 by Hogrefe Publishing
www.hogrefe.com

The authors and publisher have made every effort to ensure that the information contained in this text is in accord with the current state of scientific knowledge, recommendations, and practice at the time of publication. In spite of this diligence, errors cannot be completely excluded. Also, due to changing regulations and continuing research, information may become outdated at any point. The authors and publisher disclaim any responsibility for any consequences which may follow from the use of information presented in this book.

Registered trademarks are not noted specifically as such in this publication. The use of descriptive names, registered names, and trademarks does not imply, even in the absence of a specific statement, that such names are exempt from the relevant protective laws and regulations and therefore free for general use.

Cover image: © HaizhanZheng – iStock.com

PUBLISHING OFFICES

USA:	Hogrefe Publishing Corporation, 44 Merrimac St., Suite 207, Newburyport, MA 01950 Phone 978 255 3700; E-mail customersupport@hogrefe.com
EUROPE:	Hogrefe Publishing GmbH, Merkelstr. 3, 37085 Göttingen, Germany Phone +49 551 99950 0, Fax +49 551 99950 111; E-mail publishing@hogrefe.com

SALES & DISTRIBUTION

USA:	Hogrefe Publishing, Customer Services Department, 30 Amberwood Parkway, Ashland, OH 44805 Phone 800 228 3749, Fax 419 281 6883; E-mail customersupport@hogrefe.com
UK:	Hogrefe Publishing, c/o Marston Book Services Ltd., 160 Eastern Ave., Milton Park, Abingdon, OX14 4SB Phone +44 1235 465577, Fax +44 1235 465556; E-mail direct.orders@marston.co.uk
EUROPE:	Hogrefe Publishing, Merkelstr. 3, 37085 Göttingen, Germany Phone +49 551 99950 0, Fax +49 551 99950 111; E-mail publishing@hogrefe.com

OTHER OFFICES

CANADA:	Hogrefe Publishing Corporation, 82 Laird Drive, East York, Ontario, M4G 3V1
SWITZERLAND:	Hogrefe Publishing, Länggass-Strasse 76, 3012 Bern

No part of this book may be reproduced, stored in a retrieval system or transmitted, in any form or by any means, electronic, mechanical, photocopying, microfilming, recording or otherwise, without written permission from the publisher.

Printed and bound in the USA

ISBN 978-0-88937-507-9 (print) · ISBN 978-1-61676-507-1 (PDF) · ISBN 978-1-61334-507-8 (EPUB)
https://doi.org/10.1027/00507-000

Acknowledgments

We would like to acknowledge our longtime community partners and collaborators who have unwaveringly supported the research that forms the foundation of this book, including our friends and colleagues at the Downtown Emergency Service Center, Evergreen Treatment Services – REACH program, the People's Harm Reduction Alliance, Pioneer Human Services at the Dutch Shisler Sobering Support Center, Seattle/King County Public Health, Seattle/King County Behavioral Health and Recovery Division, Catholic Housing Services, among others. We also acknowledge the support of our institutions, the University of Washington School of Medicine and Washington State University, as well as our funders at the National Institutes of Health and the Alcohol and Drug Abuse Institute.

We would also like to thank our longtime consultants, colleagues, and collaborators in this research, including Dr. Patt Denning, Dr. Mark Duncan, Dr. Bonnie Duran, Noah Fay, T. Ron Jackson, Shilo Jama, Dr. Mary Larimer, Jeannie Little, Daniel Malone, Dr. Joseph Merrill, Dr. Lonnie Nelson, Dr. Michele Peake-Andrasik, Dr. Richard K. Ries, Dr. Andrew Saxon, and Dr. Brian Smart. We thank our staff, students, and trainees at the Harm Reduction Research and Treatment (HaRRT) Center, without whom we could not have conducted the research that has informed this book. We especially thank Emily Taylor, our senior research coordinator, for her hard work and dedication coordinating multiple treatment trials over the past decade. We also acknowledge the work of the clinicians and administrators of the harm reduction treatment (HaRT) track at Harborview Medical Center many of whom kindly reviewed this manuscript.

We honor the memory of the late Dr. G. Alan Marlatt, who entrusted us with some projects he held dear, whose trailblazing work inspired our efforts, and for whose mentorship we will always be grateful. We also thank Dr. William R. Miller for his work on the spirit of motivational interviewing, which has deeply informed our work as clinicians, and for his help in drawing parallels and distinctions between motivational interviewing and harm reduction treatment. We thank Dr. Linda Sobell for her astute editorial help. We are also deeply grateful to her and Dr. Mark Sobell for their early and courageous work in non-abstinence-based treatment, natural recovery, guided self-change, and more nuanced measurements of substance use, all of which likewise formed a strong foundation for this book.

We acknowledge and hope to honor in this work the immeasurable contributions of our various community advisory board members and community consultants over the years, as well as the hundreds of patients, clients, and research participants that contributed their experiences to this work. We especially honor the memory of Joey Stanton, beloved community consultant and mentor, whom we cite in this book. We thank Lovella Black Bear and Grover "Will" Williams, who are longtime community advisory board members who contributed their words and to whom we are grateful for every co-learning moment. Many community members – research participants, clients, community advisory board members – have told us over the years that they simply hoped their own experiences could help someone else in need and could help their communities heal. We believe they have.

Finally, we dedicate this book to our families, who have their own long and complicated histories with substances, substance use and SUD, and for whose future we are fighting.

Contents

Acknowledgments v
Preface ix

1	**Description**	1
1.1	Terminology and Definitions	2
1.1.1	Harm Reduction Heartset Is Foundational	2
1.1.2	Harm Reduction Mindset Is Pragmatic	2
1.1.3	Harm Reduction Across Ecological Systems	3
1.2	Applying Harm Reduction in Clinical Work	3
1.2.1	Accepting Substance Use Is Here to Stay	3
1.2.2	Acknowledging Reasons for Clients' Use	3
1.2.3	Recognizing Substance-Related Harm Is Shaped by Systems	4
1.2.4	Supporting Clients' Own Steps Toward Harm Reduction ...	6
1.2.5	Working Toward Social Justice and Racial Equity	7
1.3	Rationale for Harm Reduction	8
1.3.1	Abstinence-Only Approaches Are Disempowering	8
1.3.2	Abstinence-Only Approaches Do Not Consistently Engage .	10
1.3.3	Harm Reduction Approaches Are Effective	11
1.4	The Harm Reduction Treatment Model	12
1.5	Related and Foundational Treatment Models	14
1.5.1	"Controlled Drinking"	15
1.5.2	Brief Interventions in Health Care Settings	16
1.5.3	Personalized Normative Feedback Interventions	16
1.5.4	Motivational Interviewing	17
1.5.5	Guided Self-Change	17
1.5.6	Harm Reduction Psychotherapy	18
1.6	Conclusions	19
2	**Theories and Models**	20
2.1	Pharmacological Treatment for Harm Reduction	20
2.2	Behavioral Harm Reduction Treatment	22
2.2.1	HaRT Mindset	23
2.2.2	HaRT Heartset	25
2.2.3	HaRT Components	26
2.3	What HaRT Is *Not*	29
3	**Assessment and Treatment Indications**	32
3.1	Treatment Indication	32
3.2	Preparation for HaRT	33
3.2.1	Reflecting On and Readying Your Practice Setting	33
3.2.2	Preparing to Navigate Systems For and With Clients	36

3.3	Assessment of HaRT Efficacy on Key Outcomes	40
3.3.1	Assessment of Safer-Use Strategies and Harm Reduction Goal Setting	40
3.3.2	Assessment of Substance Use Outcomes	42
3.3.3	Lab Testing and Biomarkers	43
3.3.4	Measures of QoL Outcomes	44
3.3.5	Measures for Utilization and Cost Analysis	44
3.3.6	Treatment Integrity Materials and Measures	45
4	**HaRT Implementation**	**46**
4.1	Method of Approach	46
4.1.1	HaRT Mindset	46
4.1.2	HaRT Heartset	51
4.1.3	HaRT Components and Their Integration in Initial and Follow-Up Sessions	63
4.1.4	Auxiliary HaRT Components	78
4.2	HaRT Efficacy and Prognosis	84
4.2.1	Behavioral Harm Reduction Treatment for AUD	84
4.2.2	Combined Pharmacotherapy and Behavioral Treatment	86
4.3	Problems in Carrying Out the Approaches	86
4.4	Diversity Issues	88
5	**Afterword**	**90**
6	**Case Vignettes**	**91**
7	**Further Reading**	**95**
8	**References**	**97**
9	**Appendix: Tools and Resources**	**108**

Preface

We are writing this preface over 2 years into the global COVID-19 pandemic, which hit the US with force in early 2020. The past 2 years have been both a harrowing and a heady time in our nation's history, full of seismic shifts toward healing and justice, as well as heartbreaking losses and setbacks. The field of substance use treatment and research has been a part of this picture. The pandemic ushered in record-breaking rates of morbidity and mortality, disproportionately impacting communities of color, people with disabilities, and older people. For many, however, the toll went beyond the infection and its proximal sequelae. As the psychological impacts of the pandemic took hold, overdose deaths and alcohol-related deaths due to accidents and liver disease spiked in unprecedented ways.

Fortunately, just in time to meet this challenge, high-ranking government officials in the US have warmed to harm reduction as national policy. For the first time in history, the White House has formally embraced harm reduction: The Biden–Harris administration's inaugural National Drug Control Strategy centers harm reduction as essential to "keep people alive" and "engage and build trust with people who use drugs" (White House et al., 2022). The definition of "recovery" from the National Institute on Alcohol Abuse and Alcoholism was recently expanded beyond abstinence to include remission from symptoms of alcohol use disorder, cessation of "heavy drinking," and improvements in biopsychosocial functioning and quality of life (Hagman et al., 2022). National leaders in substance use treatment, policy, and research funding recently defined the concept of *preaddiction* to introduce more nuance into the diagnosis of substance use disorder and more approachable pathways for primary and secondary prevention (McLellan et al., 2022). As harm reduction researchers and clinicians, we appreciate these steps.

Of course, people who use substances, and their families and their communities, have been engaging in ways to reduce harm long before these recent steps, often in the face of government inaction and even persecution. The specific term "harm reduction" has, over the past 4 decades, come to be most closely associated with grassroots activism and public health efforts to reduce harm associated with substance use and sexual behaviors, particularly in response to the HIV/AIDS crisis of the 80s and 90s. We acknowledge the importance of the vast and diverse harm reduction work done in communities, across professional disciplines, and around the world. For this reason, we want to be clear that this book will address just one narrow aspect of the larger field of harm reduction. Namely, we are US-based and Western-trained substance use treatment clinicians who are writing a psychotherapeutic manual on an evidence-based harm reduction treatment practice developed with and for people who use substances.

With this focus in mind, harm reduction for substance use is a set of compassionate and pragmatic approaches to reduce substance-related harm and improve quality of life for people who use substances, their families, and their communities. The modern harm reduction movement has been underpinned by strong grassroots efforts that have often been led by people who use substances and have been marginalized within the system. In our roles as researchers and clinicians, we have sought to positively contribute to harm reduction, while being mindful of the concerns about governmental, public health, and academic appropriation of the work. We have engaged in long-term collaborations with community members and community-based agencies to share resources, co-learn, cocreate, implement, evaluate, and disseminate the work you are reading about here.

This book, *Harm Reduction Treatment for Substance Use,* is laid out similarly to others in the *Advances in Psychotherapy – Evidence-Based Practice* series. In Chapter 1, we provide definitions, scientific rationale, and historically relevant models that informed the development of HaRT, and in Chapter 2, we detail its underpinning theoretical tenets. In Chapter 3, we review treatment indications and practice preparation for HaRT. We also review psychometrically sound assessment tools we have used in research trials and clinical practice to inform, guide, and evaluate our application of HaRT. Early in Chapter 4, we describe the implementation of HaRT in outpatient psychotherapy and community-based settings. Then we share HaRT's evidence base, challenges in its application, and its placement in cultural context. We close with two case vignettes in Chapter 5 and provide further readings that expand on harm reduction treatment in Chapter 6. In the Appendices, we have provided measures and worksheets to facilitate application of HaRT in clinical practice.

As we share information about HaRT for your consideration, we want to acknowledge and thank the grassroots activists and thought leaders who have spent decades fighting for harm reduction treatment, programming, and policy, often at great risk to themselves, to help their communities survive and thrive. We are thus donating any royalties we receive from this book to community-based harm reduction agencies, from whom we have learned so much.

1
Description

We did not start out as harm reductionists. Seema L. Clifasefi was originally trained, not as a clinician, but as a cognitive and experimental psychologist, designing experiments to manipulate participants' memories and experiences. These studies were undergirded by researcher-driven theories about others' realities, testing the effects of alcohol and alcohol placebos on cognitive and perceptual processes, such as eyewitness memory, inattentional blindness, and false memories. Susan E. Collins, with a recovery history of her own and the intergenerational experience of substance use disorder (SUD), spent time in the 12-step community, diligently learned the pantheon of treatments that encourage people to change in counselor-sanctioned ways, and stood in bathrooms with rubber gloves on, collecting drug toxicology samples, and writing letters to judges.

Instead, the harm reduction movement changed us slowly over time, reshaping our practices, our careers, and our lives. We were changed by conversations with our mentors, including G. Alan Marlatt, PhD, Mary Larimer, PhD, Patt Denning, PhD, Jeannie Little, LICSW, and Linda Sobell, PhD, trailblazers in drinking moderation and harm reduction approaches. We were changed by the teachings of community members who had to "bang on the table" to be heard in service settings (Collins et al., 2018), of front-line case managers who told us that harm reduction is the "only thing that works" (Collins, Clifasefi, Dana, et al., 2012), of activists organizing for users' rights and providing services to their own communities – the Junkiebond, VOCAL, National Harm Reduction Coalition, Chicago Recovery Alliance, People's Harm Reduction Alliance, Urban Survivor's Union, among others. These teachings made us deeply reflect on our own frustrations with our belief systems, our institutions, our research, and our clinical practices.

We believe this change for us is also happening for many others in our field. Perhaps it reflects a larger sea change that is sweeping across our scientific disciplines, our clinical practices, and the larger collective culture in the US. In substance use and mental health counseling, more narrowly, clinicians, therapists, and counselors are increasingly aware of and learning from grassroots harm reduction movements and from their own clients (Collins, Clifasefi, Andrasik, et al., 2012; Hawk et al., 2017). As harm reduction clinicians, we must support these grassroots efforts without co-opting them, and we need to ask ourselves what we, in our professional identities, can offer to this movement. In response, we wrote this book to describe the evidence-based harm reduction treatment modality we have spent the last decade codeveloping, implementing, and evaluating, together with communities marginalized by substance-related harm.

1.1 Terminology and Definitions

Harm reduction approaches do not require abstinence but aim to reduce harm and improve quality of life

As applied to substance use intervention, the umbrella term "harm reduction" refers to a compassionate stance and a set of pragmatic strategies that minimize substance-related harm and enhance QoL for people who use substances, their families, and their communities (Collins et al., 2011). As its name implies, harm reduction breaks with traditional abstinence-based approaches in that its focus is on minimizing harm, and it does not require or even particularly elevate abstinence or use reduction as ultimate goals (Heather, 2006). While we appreciate the contributions of abstinence-based approaches as important and effective recovery pathways for some, we believe harm reduction approaches are necessary additions to the spectrum of care to ensure greater treatment reach, engagement, and effectiveness.

1.1.1 Harm Reduction Heartset Is Foundational

The harm reduction heartset is culturally humble and compassionate

As defined above, harm reduction can be described as a set of strategies; however, it is the culturally humble and compassionate spirit or *harm reduction heartset* with which strategies are applied that is essential. In fact, this heartset should drive the nature of more concrete interventions and the way they are implemented and thereby received by the community. Of course, we are not the first ones to say this. Dave Purchase, the late and great founding director of the North America Syringe Exchange Network (NASEN) and the Tacoma Needle Exchange noted that harm reduction is more "an attitude" than a fixed set of approaches (Marlatt, 1998b, p. 6). Handing out clean syringes constitutes a fairly concrete harm reduction intervention, but Purchase knew the most important part was *how* he set up his program to center people who use substances, *how* he handed out syringes with nonjudgment, and *how* he was in community with love, humility, and compassion in this work.

1.1.2 Harm Reduction Mindset Is Pragmatic

Pragmatism means meeting clients where they are at in their communities and in their motivation for change

Adopting a *harm reduction mindset* is pragmatic for those of us seeking to work with the entire spectrum of people who use substances. After all, it is substance-related harm that drives the diagnosis of substance use disorder in the *Diagnostic and Statistical Manual of Mental Disorders*, 5th edition (DSM-5). Pragmatism also drives harm reduction clinicians' additional focus on QoL. Our research has shown that people who use substances are striving to meet their basic needs and engage in meaningful activities, just as much if not more than changing their substance use (Fentress et al., 2021). This same research has shown that a clinical focus that prioritizes both what people want to leave behind (i.e., substance-related harm) *and* what they want to move toward (e.g., engaging in meaningful activities, fulfilling basic needs) is associated with positive treatment outcomes (Fentress et al., 2021).

1.1.3 Harm Reduction Across Ecological Systems

Thinking more systemically (Bronfenbrenner, 1979), harm reduction approaches for substance use may be, and are, applied at various levels. Taking the widest lens, macrosystem-level approaches comprise policy changes (e.g., decriminalizing, legalizing, and regulating substance use; Marlatt & Witkiewitz, 2010) or large-scale provision of high-coverage, combined intervention programs (e.g., comprehensive medication for opioid use disorder [MOUD] plus syringe programs plus antiretroviral therapy; Degenhardt et al., 2010). At the population level, harm reduction can take the form of public health messaging and public service announcements (e.g., the 1983 "friends don't let friends drive drunk" campaign from the Ad Council). At the community level, harm reduction approaches are often applied within higher-risk communities to reduce risks for that community, as well as the surrounding environment (e.g., low-barrier, non-abstinence-based "Housing First," needle and syringe programs, safer consumption sites). Finally, harm reduction at the individual level encompasses treatment, counseling, or other one-on-one or group healing approaches (Collins et al., 2011).

1.2 Applying Harm Reduction in Clinical Work

Because clinicians, psychotherapists, and counselors are most active in their professional roles on the individual level of intervention, we focus in this book on an evidence-based psychotherapeutic or counseling treatment protocol that we call *harm reduction treatment for substance use disorder* (HaRT). However, before we focus on that individual level of harm reduction, we will explore the tenets of the broader harm reduction movement and their relevance for our clinical practice.

1.2.1 Accepting Substance Use Is Here to Stay

Substance use has existed for millennia as an essential human behavior (Guerra-Doce, 2015). In our modern societies, one can surmise that most people are engaged in some kind of substance use on a regular basis. (For example, did you have your morning coffee or tea today?) We have thus concluded that it is neither an efficient nor an effective way to spend our time as clinicians trying to eradicate this long-standing human behavior. We are better positioned to do what we can today to help people and their communities reduce substance-related harm.

Focus shift from eradicating substance use to supporting harm reduction and improving QoL

1.2.2 Acknowledging Reasons for Clients' Use

In contrast to some abstinence-based ideologies (e.g., Alcoholics Anonymous, 2008), we assert that substance use is not "irrational." While we acknowledge substance-related harm, we also acknowledge the real and valid reasons our

Clinicians should be open to learning about the important reasons clients use substances

clients use (e.g., attaining and maintaining a sense of physical and psychological safety and comfort, cognitive focus, relaxation, enjoyment, and social benefits; Collins et al., 2013; Collins, Kirouac, et al., 2014; Collins, Taylor, et al., 2018). Our research has indicated that substance use is simply one way people seek to serve their overarching QoL goals (Fentress et al., 2021), which cross-cultural studies show are founded on relatively universal human goals (Grouzet et al., 2005). Recent mainstream books on drug use and harm reduction have served to elevate these perspectives (Hart, 2021; Szalavitz, 2021).

Recognizing the reasons for our clients' use has important implications for our clinical and counseling work. First off, it just makes sense to understand why our clients use substances; it helps us better understand the full clinical picture. Second, it also shows we accept our clients' perceived reality and their whole self, which conveys unconditional positive regard and strengthens the therapeutic bond. Next, it creates a safe space for clients to openly discuss their substance use. Creating an environment in which our clients feel comfortable discussing their use is essential so we can conduct an accurate substance use and mental health assessment and envision a safe and helpful treatment plan. Finally, it allows us to fully engage the tools of HaRT but also other psychotherapeutic modalities. For example, if we understand what our clients are getting out of their substance use (e.g., physical relaxation, psychological coping, supporting socializing), we are better positioned to codevelop with them ways to get what they want out of their use while minimizing risk of harm to themselves and their communities. Similarly, we might also help them consider obtaining these perceived benefits in other ways (e.g., sports, mindfulness-based strategies, finding other means of socializing).

The opposite is also true. If we do not acknowledge that people have positive experiences with substances and thus do not ask about what people get out of their substance use, we are missing vitally important clinical information, which will negatively impact our ability to help our clients.

1.2.3 Recognizing Substance-Related Harm Is Shaped by Systems

Societally shaped beliefs and values around substance use can both build community and marginalize individuals

We often talk about substance use and substance-related harm as if it were fully individually determined. We reify SUD as something that resides within the individual. We must, however, acknowledge that substance use patterns, substance-related harm, and SUD are shaped heavily by larger familial, community, commercial, socioeconomic, and even geopolitical factors. Taking a more sweeping historical view: What substances are used via what modes and for what purpose has changed dramatically across cultures and across time. What is considered socially acceptable or unacceptable use, or what is considered legal or illicit use, are likewise socially and temporally dependent, and yet these social constructs in any given time and place have real consequences that shape individuals' use and experience of substance-related harm – their social capital, their child custody, their incarceration, their job stability (see Box 1 for an example).

> **Box 1**
> **The Intersection of Anti-Black Racism, Classism, and Drug Laws**
>
> In 1986, Len Bias, a talented Black college basketball player, died of an overdose after using powder cocaine and alcohol. The disinformation spread in the aftermath: the falsehood that Bias's overdose was due to crack cocaine, the myth that crack cocaine was more dangerous, addictive, and violence-inducing than powder cocaine, and the exaggerated fear that youth and unborn babies were particularly susceptible to its effects. These myths have been debunked. Crack and powder cocaine are pharmacologically the same, but crack is less expensive to produce and was thus more widely available in lower-income urban areas. It is also important to note that, while past-year prevalence of crack cocaine use is more common among Blacks, lifetime crack cocaine use and past-year cocaine use overall (including the more expensive powder cocaine) is more prevalent in non-Latinx Whites. Nonetheless, the media frenzy around Bias's overdose, the proliferation of fear-based disinformation, and race- and class-based scapegoating propelled the swift passage of the Anti-Drug Abuse Act of 1986, which arbitrarily set minimum federal prison sentences for crack versus powder cocaine to a 100:1 ratio. That means that distribution of 5 g of crack led to the same sentencing as 500 g of powder cocaine. In 2010, this law was changed, but the ratio remains inequitable at 18:1. The upshot? Despite the fact that the prevalence of cocaine use was and continues to be highest among White, non-Latinx people, Black people continue – even 35 years later – to comprise the majority of federal incarcerations for cocaine-related crimes. Anti-Black racism and classism shaped federal drug laws that led to vastly disproportionate and intergenerational harm for Black families and communities, and particularly for those in lower-income urban areas.

Consider even more discretely defined constructs that we clinicians know well, such as the definition of alcohol use disorder (AUD) according to the DSM-5. The definition is clear and adhered to like a checklist, determining treatment access, billable services, and diagnoses that follow clients across health care systems. However, it is important to remember that this definition has changed every decade or 2 since the manual's first, heavily psychodynamic-flavored first edition. For example, in 2013, everything we knew about the defining aspects of, say, "alcohol abuse" or "alcohol dependence" in the *Diagnostic and Statistical Manual of Mental Disorders*, 4th edition, text revision (DSM-IV-TR) changed, when the DSM-5's "alcohol use disorder – mild, moderate, severe" took its place. The fact that such labels can and do shift overnight without our clients' input and without any change in their actual experiences and behaviors is jolting when we consider how such labels impact clients' access to help, treatment course, and larger life trajectories from job prospects to child custody. Thus, these larger, systemic factors are deeply impactful in shaping individuals' experiences with substances and, the research shows us, can be more predictive of individuals' experiences of substance-related harm than their own individual substance use (Collins, 2016).

In acknowledging that substance use and the experience of substance-related harm are so heavily externally influenced, we acknowledge as a corollary that substance use is not the client, and the client is not their substance use. We are, for example, daughters, mothers, sisters, teachers, scientists, therapists – and we are just talking about ourselves!

> Labels like "addict," "alcoholic," and "substance abuser" are negatively impactful

There is, however, a more pressing clinical need to avoid labels, which is a stance likewise taken in other person-centered treatments (Miller & Rollnick, 2013). When we label people as "addicts" or "alcoholics," we reduce them to just one behavior they engage in, which does not leave room for their personhood and their strengths. Further, while some clients may embrace such labels for themselves, research has indicated that clinicians' application of such labels can be punitive, stigmatizing, and discourage treatment engagement for clients (Kulesza et al., 2013). Even seemingly small changes in terminology (e.g., referring to an individual as "a substance abuser" vs. "having a substance use disorder") can inspire a more punitive mindset in clinicians (Kelly & Westerhoff, 2010). Thus, harm reduction clinicians must advocate for the use of person-first language and the eradication of stigmatizing labels (Earnshaw, 2020).

1.2.4 Supporting Clients' Own Steps Toward Harm Reduction

> "Tough love" from clinicians is more hurtful than helpful to people who use substances

Harm reduction clinicians support people who use substances to reduce substance-related harm – for themselves, their families, and their communities. We must be aware, however, that only clients can drive their own behavior – maintaining their existing use patterns, moving toward increased harm, or reduced harm. We thus strive to avoid "tough love" or confrontational approaches, which when stemming from a "doctor-knows-best" assumption, can have iatrogenic effects (White & Miller, 2007). More pragmatic than cliché, dropping the "tough" out of the "tough love" approach allows us to spend our clinical time simply loving our clients instead of distrusting, berating, bouncing, or resenting them. In our own clinical experiences and our qualitative research, this open and compassionate stance facilitates greater mutual respect, trust, and co-learning (Collins, Jones, et al., 2016; Collins, Orfaly, et al., 2018; Nelson et al., 2022). It elevates and affirms clients, bolstering their ability and self-efficacy to forge their own recovery pathway.

Similar to other psychotherapeutic approaches, the client-led aspect of harm reduction requires that we, as harm reduction clinicians, are aware of our values and that we ensure we are not imposing them on our clients. This task is often more challenging than it sounds, because our professional values, in particular, are often formed in the early days of our training and baked into our treatment systems. We are often not consciously aware of them and can often not find citations for them; they simply *are*. We are most often implicitly expecting clients to perform in accordance with our treatment standards and program expectations, and these standards are often written by White, male physicians with high socioeconomic status. As harm reduction clinicians, we must interrogate and perhaps set aside these value systems that are imposed by our cultural reference points, professions, trainings, and programs, to truly honor the value system of the person sitting across from us. That also means being open to the power of, and enthusiastically affirming, any positive change – even if it seems incremental (e.g., safer injection vs. total abstinence) within our traditional professional values systems.

1.2.5 Working Toward Social Justice and Racial Equity

A few years ago, Susan E. Collins was asked by the National Institute on Alcohol Abuse and Alcoholism to review the scientific literature and report on the associations between alcohol use and socioeconomic status (Collins, 2016). The most consistent finding represented across studies and cultures all around the world was the fact that people from dominant parts of a given society – in the US that often translates to White, male, cisgender, heterosexual, high socioeconomic status, high educational status – could and often did drink larger amounts of alcohol and experienced, by comparison, less severe consequences than people from minoritized or marginalized communities (e.g., People of Color; people who are socioeconomically marginalized; womxn; and lesbian, gay, bisexual, transgender, questioning and/or queer, intersex, asexual, two-spirit, and other identities [LGBTQIA2+]).

> People who are minoritized and marginalized are disproportionately impacted by substance-related harm

This finding is not to imply that people from dominant parts of society are protected from *any* experience of substance-related harm; substance use can engender very severe harm across various strata in society. It does mean that minoritized and marginalized groups within a given society have a greater experience of substance-related harm that is not fully accounted for by level of use. Those most impacted in our practices will be People of Color, people who are socioeconomically marginalized, people from rural communities, womxn, LGBTQIA2+, and children. We see that harm morph into systemic, long-term, and devastating effects, such as mass incarceration, where systems have shunted entire generations of people into the interlocking systems of oppression of the criminal justice, prison, and foster systems.

It is necessary but not sufficient to acknowledge these systems inequities. We must also advocate on behalf of clients and connect them with user-led, grassroots, and community groups (e.g., VOCAL, National Drug User's Union) that build community capacity in advocacy and activism. As harm reduction clinicians, we must also acknowledge our role in the interlocking systems of oppression and strive to do better. There are some movements calling for the abolition of Western, Eurocentric counseling fields (Toronto Abolition Convergence, 2020), and we are actively interrogating our practices, our fields (psychology and social work), and learning more about abolition as a way forward. However, until more effective, well-funded, and culturally aligned systems are in place, many of us will continue to do our best to support our clients within the existing systems.

We must, however, be responsive to the core demands of these movements. Both individually and organizationally – we must examine our own power and privilege and how that impacts our service provision within our treatment systems. For example, anytime we write a letter to a judge or a probation officer that our client has provided a positive urine toxicology test, we are exposing our clients to risk of incarceration or other punitive measures meted out by the criminal justice system. We must resist systemic pressures to engage in behaviors that contribute to mass incarceration. We must respect

> As harm reduction clinicians, we must critically examine and check our own power and privilege

our clients', families', and communities' autonomy and ensure they lead the work we do in our sessions. Clients are understood to be the experts on and the decision makers about their own pathways. We, as harm reduction clinicians, honor their goals and uplift their preferred pathways to these goals. In sum, we need to carefully consider and dampen the potential negative downstream effect of our work and our systems. And, now here we are, full circle back to where we started, talking about harm reduction and how we need to honor its grassroots and center the voices and interests of people who use substances.

1.3 Rationale for Harm Reduction

As clinicians, we need to be clear regarding our rationale for moving from an abstinence-based to a harm reduction approach. This decision can have a big impact on our potential client base; outreach efforts; intake evaluations, diagnostics, and outcome assessments; case conceptualizations; treatment planning; treatment reach; potential funding; and interactions within systems of care. We will discuss what this move entails, more specifically in Chapters 3 and 4. In the following section, we explain our scientifically and clinically based reasoning for this move.

1.3.1 Abstinence-Only Approaches Are Disempowering

Many people find the abstinence-based treatment system to be disempowering

Many years ago, Susan E. Collins walked into the breakroom of a substance use treatment agency where our research team was conducting relapse prevention groups for a randomized controlled trial. There was a sign on the wall of the breakroom, so it was something the employees of the agency could see, but clients could not. The sign read, "Our clients are very sick, and they often lie to us."

This messaging has long been recognized as an amalgam of what we call the medical or disease model ("our clients are very sick") and the moral model ("they often lie to us") that forms the basis of our modern understanding of substance use and SUD in the US (Marlatt & Gordon, 1985). The medical or disease model, championed early on by Benjamin Rush and later by E. M. Jellinek (Marlatt et al., 1993), defines SUD as a "chronic, relapsing brain disease" (Leshner, 1997; National Institute on Drug Abuse, 2008). The moral model, derived from early Christian temperance movements (Marlatt et al., 1993), and further developed through the 12-step movement, suggests this "disease" is so insidious, it even causes lesions on one's moral character ("character defects"; Alcoholics Anonymous, 2008). It drives people to do bad things, like lie to us, their physicians, counselors, clinicians, and case managers. Following through to the logical conclusion of this combined medical and moral model, substance use is the cause for clients' medical problems and moral failings. Given the latter, they need professionals to point that out and guide them toward the appropriate goal, which is achieving and maintaining abstinence (Heilig et al., 2021; National Institute on Drug

Abuse, 2008). The corollary is that, by not prohibiting substance use and by supporting clients' choice about their substance use goals, non-abstinence-based approaches may "enable" or facilitate continued, harmful drinking (Denning & Little, 2012).

At the bottom of that sign in the breakroom, however, someone had scrawled in pen, "And sometimes they tell the truth." That act of defiance shows a move away from the absolute nature of the messaging that preceded it. It is the kind of nuanced understanding that we must embrace to support our clients in incremental change toward harm reduction.

> **Clinical Vignette 1**
> Susan E. Collins's Personal Experience With Tough Love
>
> If you come from a place of privilege wherein you have been able to maintain some control over the flow of your life, we would ask you: Have you ever lied to your doctor or an employer about smoking, or how much you are drinking or have used drugs?
>
> Susan shares: "I did until I had health problems related to my substance use that were undeniable to the doctors from whom I sought help. I was sat down for 'the talk' and was told I was an 'alcoholic.' I felt the shame flood my body, and I argued back: 'No, I am not. 'Alcoholic' has not been a diagnostic category since the DSM-II.' The physician looked at me with pity and responded that I was 'in denial' before he told me I needed to stop drinking for the sake of my family and my health and go to abstinence-based treatment. Despite my extreme privilege in that situation, I felt shame, anger, resentment, and entrapment, likely similar to what my clients had always felt in the treatment systems I was working in. Unlike for other medical diagnoses, substance use disorder is not managed collaboratively such that clients can contemplate a clinician's diagnosis, ask questions, get a second opinion, or consider multiple options for recovery goals and pathways. At worst, there is dire punishment (e.g., denied liver transplant, threat of imprisonment, loss of child custody). At best, there is this disconnected emergency department doctor's 'tough love,' which, when one is on the receiving end, does not really feel like love at all."

Yet, as harm reduction clinicians we must take this nuanced stance a step further. Considering our interlocking systems of oppression, of which the treatment system is a key component, it impossible for our clients to *not* lie to us (see Clinical Vignette 1 for one of our perspectives). This assertion might sound shocking, so let us take a moment to look at a routine aspect of our substance use treatment system. We clinicians feel compelled, and often are compelled through our systems' policies and financial contracts with other entities, to be informants on our clients. We routinely conduct complex, intrusive, and humiliating toxicology assay procedures (e.g., observing clients as they provide urine samples, cutting clients' hair) and send toxicology reports and letters to nonclinicians – employers, child protective services, courts, and probation and parole officers – detailing our clients' substance use as well as treatment attendance, plans, and progress. Somewhere along the way we were converted from well-intentioned healers charged with protecting privacy and confidentiality, to proxy judge, jury, and jailer. We do not talk about this as clinicians, but perhaps some of us appreciated the sense of systemic or personal power this gave us when confronted with the real pain and hardship of our clients and a sense of powerlessness to help them. We must also confront darker potential motives: Perhaps we enjoyed controlling the fates of others.

In any case, we have given clients no choice but to lie to us to survive in the system: They do not want to lose their access to treatment, their jobs, custody of their children, their freedom from incarceration. That sounds pretty reasonable. On the other side, we clinicians have been empowered by the interlocking systems of oppression to take away the things they value most, armed with our urine cups and a stroke of our pen.

1.3.2 Abstinence-Only Approaches Do Not Consistently Engage

Although some thought leaders in the field are warming to alternative end points for recovery (e.g., Hagman et al., 2022), abstinence is still the widely accepted and largely unquestioned norm in substance use treatment practice. Unfortunately, abstinence-based treatment fails to optimally engage some of the most marginalized people who use substances in our communities (e.g., people who experience homelessness). Although studies suggest that abstinence-based treatments for people experiencing homelessness are associated with modest improvements in alcohol outcomes (Hwang et al., 2006; Smith et al., 1998; Zerger, 2002), these improvements are only experienced by the few who are engaged and retained in treatment (Zerger, 2002). The few studies addressing the topic show that a minority of people experiencing homelessness start treatment (15–28%; Rosenheck et al., 1998; Wenzel et al., 2001), and even fewer complete it (2.5–33% ; Orwin et al., 1999). A National Institute on Alcohol Abuse and Alcoholism review of substance use treatment programs in the US showed that treatment engagement in this population decreased as program demands – particularly abstinence from substances – increased (Orwin et al., 1999).

More recent studies have indicated potential reasons for these findings. In our prior research, participants indicated they were not interested in abstinence-based approaches (Clifasefi et al., 2016; Collins, Clifasefi, Dana, et al., 2012; Collins, Jones, et al., 2016). This finding was not based in people's disinterest in treatment. In one of our studies, participants reported having experienced a mean of 16 abstinence-based treatment episodes in their lifetimes (Larimer et al., 2009). Perhaps it goes without saying that if our abstinence-based, relapse prevention treatment system were consistently effective for this population, participants would not have reported attending abstinence-based treatment a mean of 16 times. They would not have been sitting in the interview with us in their supportive housing program for people with severe AUD. Far from disinterest, these participants were scientists running the odds of a positive future treatment outcome – the 17th time around. They logically determined their odds were not great. Thus, their lack of treatment engagement was not due to a disinterest in feeling better, it was due to a scientifically informed disappointment in our system's ability to help them.

These low levels of treatment engagement, interest, and positive outcomes are not, however, unique to marginalized populations and people who are most severely impacted by substance-related harm. It also holds for people with SUD more generally. The yearly National Survey on Drug Use and Health of the Substance Abuse and Mental Health Services Administration (SAMHSA), which is conducted with a large, randomly selected sample of the general US population, has shown a similar and highly consistent pattern over the past decade. In 2021, only about 6% of the 43 million people with SUD received treatment (SAMHSA, 2022). Among those who met criteria for but did not receive treatment, 97% reported they did not need it (SAMHSA, 2022). Now, SAMHSA does not ask the obvious follow-up which is, "Why did you feel that way?" Or better yet, "Why did you not go to treatment?" But for whatever reason, we can safely conclude that our treatment system is not desirable, relevant, accessible (or whatever else) to the vast majority of Americans it is supposed to serve.

1.3.3 Harm Reduction Approaches Are Effective

Research has established a strong evidence base for harm reduction approaches and provided viable future directions. Regarding AUD, community-based harm reduction approaches have been applied and investigated primarily within marginalized populations, including with people experiencing homelessness and AUD. Two randomized controlled trials of the HaRT approach introduced in this book, both with and without medication support, have indicated that harm reduction treatment applied at the individual level is engaging and effective in reducing alcohol use and alcohol-related harm (Collins, Clifasefi, et al., 2019; Collins, Duncan, et al., 2021). Randomized controlled trials have also established the effectiveness of the provision of immediate, permanent, low-barrier, non-abstinence-based supportive housing to people experiencing chronic homelessness. This approach, known as Housing First, has been shown to be associated with increased housing stability, decreased alcohol use and alcohol-related harm, and reductions in use of publicly funded services, such as the emergency department, jail, and emergency medical services (Malone et al., 2015; Stergiopoulos et al., 2015). Managed alcohol programs and meaningful activities programming, such as art groups, gardening, and music, have shown promising findings in nonrandomized trials and warrant further study (Collins et al., 2022; Pauly et al., 2018; Stockwell et al., 2018).

Effective across populations, substances, and levels of application

Regarding smoking, the pathway to harm reduction is relatively clear. Smoking's greatest risks are not due to nicotine or even tobacco but the *tobacco smoke being inhaled into the lungs.* Inhaling tobacco smoke is a highly effective means of distributing chemicals throughout the body that strain the cardiovascular system (e.g., carbon monoxide) and cause cancer (e.g., tobacco-specific nitrosamines and polycyclic aromatic hydrocarbons). Aside from its strong addictive properties, pure nicotine is relatively harmless to adults in the amounts usually consumed. Thus, a harm reduction approach entails replacing smoking behavior with safer means of obtaining nicotine. Although exposure to any tobacco confers greater risk than no exposure, researchers have shown that smokeless tobacco use is associated with less toxicant exposure (Chang et al., 2021) and risk for cardiovascular harm (Rezk-Hanna et al., 2022), and that switching from smoking to smokeless tobacco can reduce cardiovascular risk (Lee, 2013). Even smoking reduction is associated with reductions in cardiovascular risk factors, respiratory symptoms, incidence of lung cancer, small increases in birth weight, and increased odds of smoking cessation attempts and achievement (Begh et al., 2015; Chang et al., 2021; Pisinger & Godtfredsen, 2007). Earlier European studies indicated that even longer-term use of nicotine replacement therapy (e.g., patch, gum, lozenge) and the replacement of smoking with electronic nicotine delivery system (e.g., e-cigarettes and vaping) can be 95% safer than smoking (Nutt et al., 2014). More recently, an expansive review of the literature by the National Academies of Sciences, Engineering and Medicine (2018) confirmed that electronic nicotine delivery systems confer fewer health risks than cigarette smoking.

Regarding other drugs, harm reduction enacted at the policy and population levels has been highly effective in addressing substance-related harm. For example, drug decriminalization in Portugal has been associated with decreased criminal justice system contacts, lifetime drug use, blood-borne infection, overdose, and drug-related mortality, and it is an effective means of righting the social injustice of mass incarceration for drug-related charges (Earp et al., 2021). Regarding opioids and injection drug use more specifically, making widely available a combination of medications for opioid use disorder, needle and syringe programs, and antiretroviral therapy reduces HIV infection and overdose risks among people who use drugs (Cepeda et al., 2018; Degenhardt et al., 2010). Methadone and buprenorphine/naloxone, which are pharmaceutical-grade, controlled-dose opioids, are effective in reducing relapse to illicit opioids (Tkacz et al., 2012), and when taken regularly and over a long period of time, in preventing overdose-related mortality (Ma et al., 2019). These medications for opioid use disorder and *not* detoxification or medically supervised withdrawal now represent the gold standard for treatment.

1.4 The Harm Reduction Treatment Model

> Harm reduction treatment (HaRT) is an evidence-based application of harm reduction at the individual level

So, how do we apply the harm reduction mindset as clinicians? How can we do our part to reject complicity with systems that further marginalize people who use substances? We felt the best solution to those questions was to turn to members of the community we have regularly worked with over the past 15 years – people experiencing homelessness and SUD – and ask *them* how they would redesign substance use treatment in their own vision. We then worked alongside them to cocreate solutions, one of which we now call *harm reduction treatment* or HaRT (Figure 1).

> HaRT was cocreated and evaluated with people with SUD

HaRT was informed by harm reduction theory (Collins et al., 2011; Marlatt, 1996) and practice (Denning & Little, 2012); person-centered clinical practices (e.g., motivational interviewing and humanistic psychotherapy; Miller & Rollnick, 2013; Rogers, 1957), and by our team's 15 years of

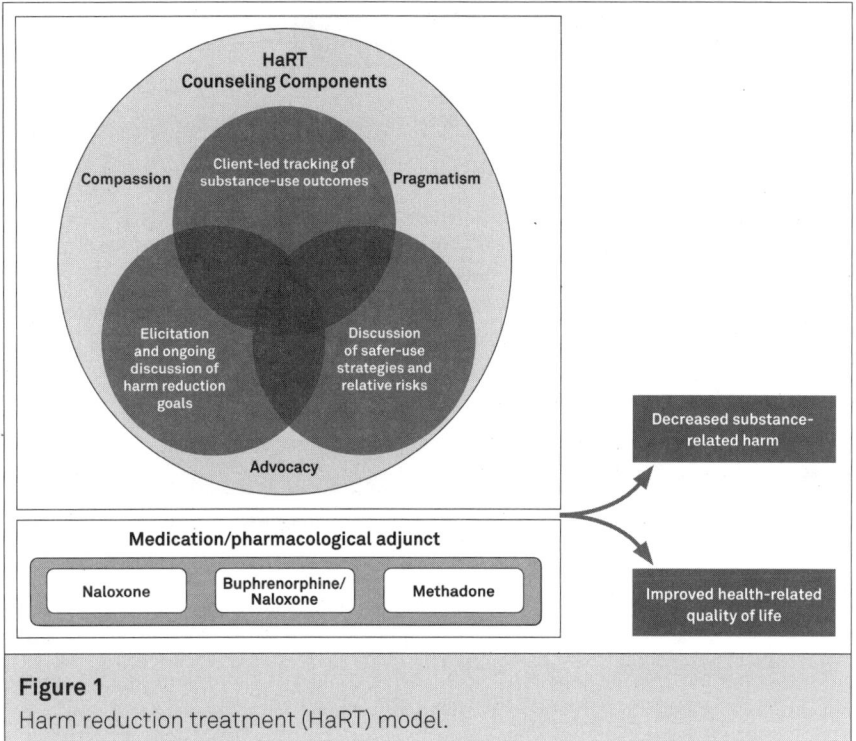

Figure 1
Harm reduction treatment (HaRT) model.

qualitative and quantitative research on the needs and preferred treatment pathways of people experiencing homelessness and SUD (Collins, Clifasefi, Dana, et al., 2012; Collins, Duncan, et al., 2015; Collins, Grazioli, et al., 2015; Collins, Jones, et al., 2016; Collins, Saxon, et al., 2014; Grazioli et al., 2014; Grazioli et al., 2015). The HaRT mindset, heartset, and components were developed by a team comprising researchers, people experiencing homelessness and AUD, and social service providers.

The HaRT *mindset* entails an application of the above-described harm reduction philosophy at the individual level. The HaRT *heartset* is a way of being with clients that entails a culturally humble, compassionate, advocacy-oriented stance and acceptance of clients wherever they fall on the spectrum of change.

Within the harm reduction mindset and heartset, HaRT further entails three concrete therapeutic components: (a) client-led tracking of substance use and harm-reduction metrics; (b) elicitation and ongoing discussion of harm-reduction goals; and (c) discussion of safer-use strategies (see Figure 1 and Figure 2). HaRT can be used in combination with medications (e.g., buprenorphine/naloxone, methadone) and other pharmacological adjuncts (e.g., vape pens) to reduce substance-related harm and improve QoL.

HaRT components: Client-led tracking of substance use and harm reduction metrics, harm reduction goal setting, and information on safer use

Client-Led Tracking of Treatment Outcomes

- Providing tailored personalized feedback on substance-use patterns (i.e., intensity and frequency of use), substance-related harm (i.e., biological markers, self-report), and quality of life (i.e., self-report).
- Focusing on improved outcomes, providing affirmations regarding reductions in high-risk substance use and substance-related harm as well as improvements in health-related quality of life (HR-QoL). Incremental changes are also affirmed. Harm reduction emphasizes the power of any positive change.
- Tracking with clients across the treatment trajectory their substance-related harm as well as other metrics they wish to track over the duration of HaRT. Counselors help clients create a graphic representation of their progress, which is updated at each session.

Elicitation and Ongoing Discussion of Harm Reduction Goals

- Eliciting clients' harm reduction goals and assessing progress made toward them. Goals might involve a focus on decreasing substance use or substance-related harm. For example, some clients might be interested in a partial or complete switchover from malt liquor to beer. Other clients might focus on achieving HR-QoL-related goals, such as climbing stairs without getting winded or starting a fitness program.
- Recording weekly harm reduction goals and collaboratively assessing at subsequent sessions whether clients have fully, partially, or not achieved their stated goals by eliciting and affirming clients' safer-use narratives.
- Helping clients break down goals into smaller, more achievable stepwise goals, and engage in troubleshooting to help clients remove barriers to goal achievement.

Discussion of Saver-Use Strategies and Relative Risks

- Providing a list of safer-use strategies as a focal point for discussing ways to stay safer and healthier, even if clients choose to use. Helping clients balance the positive and negative aspects of their use.
- Engaging clients in a conversational and ongoing discussion of scientifically based relative risks of substance-use practices, so that they make more informed decisions about their substance use.

Figure 2
Harm reduction treatment (HaRT) components.

1.5 Related and Foundational Treatment Models

The way to HaRT was paved by groundbreaking research in addiction psychology, as well as the grassroots harm reduction movement

We owe a debt of gratitude to colleagues and mentors who laid the pathway to the development of HaRT. In this section, we review historically important evidence-based interventions that have informed its development. Noting that evidence-based interventions to date have largely been developed by researchers and clinicians, we also want to acknowledge historical highlights of the modern community-led harm reduction movement (see Box 2 and Chapter 6 for suggested reading).

> **Box 2**
> **Brief History of the Modern Community-Led Harm Reduction Movement**
>
> Although this book focuses on the application of harm reduction principles within an evidence-based treatment model, this work is meant to support and not appropriate or take away from grassroots and community-led harm reduction movements around the world. In the late 70s and 80s, Nico Adriaans, a Dutch activist, scholar, and injection drug user, founded one of the early drug user unions (Junkiebond), a user-led radio show, and the first known organized syringe exchange in the world. He later contributed to harm reduction research. In 1987, New Zealand established the first nationally administered syringe exchange program, and by 1988, Australia had followed suit. Switzerland opened the first government-supported supervised consumption site in 1986, and 17 years later, Canada opened the first in North America. Medically supervised heroin administration trials started in 1992 in Europe and Canada. In 2001, Portugal became the first country to decriminalize the personal possession of all drugs. In contrast, the US government has been behind the curve on adopting harm reduction policy; early advances in harm reduction were exclusively community-led. For example, diverse, LGBTQIA2+ community-led organizations, such as Act Up, took action to address and advocate for increased attention to the HIV/AIDS crisis. People who use substances and concerned community members, such as Dave Purchase and Jon Stuen-Parker, started early syringe exchanges in the US. These often operated underground and at great risk to the community members leading this work. Only starting in 2009 could any federal funds be used to support syringe exchanges, and to this day, funds cannot be used to purchase syringes themselves. More recent community-led movements in the US have included drug-user unions advocating and organizing for harm reduction legislation, user-led medical and social service provision, housing equity, and safer consumption sites. Noting the dominance of Western entities in the modern harm reduction movement, there have been calls to decolonize harm reduction, particularly in the Global South where punitive and oppressive drug policies arrived with Western colonization. See Chapter 6: Further Reading, for suggestions on the history of harm reduction.

1.5.1 "Controlled Drinking"

In the 1970s, various research groups began exploring psychotherapeutic means of achieving lower-harm posttreatment trajectories (i.e., less heavy drinking, fewer contacts with treatment and the criminal justice system) for people with AUD. This work, conducted primarily in the US and Australia, became known at the time as *controlled drinking* (later referred to as *drinking moderation* or *low-risk drinking*) and comprised a package of behavioral modification interventions (Lovibond & Caddy, 1970; Sobell & Sobell, 1973a, 1973b). While its goals dovetailed with harm reduction, controlled drinking was based on a clinician-driven agenda and drew on aversive methods, which were common in behavioral treatment at the time. Clients received skills training in drinking moderation, engaged in self-monitoring, learned to pay attention to physical responses to different blood alcohol levels, and received aversive interventions (e.g., electrical shocks) when drinking beyond a preset amount. Findings from these early studies indicated that clients experienced less harm in their posttreatment trajectories in the controlled drinking group than in the abstinence-based treatment-as-usual group (Lovibond & Caddy, 1970; Sobell & Sobell, 1976).

As recounted by Marlatt and colleagues (1993), this early exploration of non-abstinence-based treatment options was interrupted by controversy, as popular media gave attention to unfounded claims that controlled drinking was responsible for poor and even deadly treatment outcomes. Even after these claims were debunked, there remained concern within the field that non-abstinence-based interventions were likely appropriate for at-risk drinkers but not so for people diagnosed with AUD (Sobell & Sobell, 1995). These residual concerns paired with an increasingly abstinence-oriented alcohol and drug policy environment in the 1980s and 1990s slowed the pace of research on harm reduction in the decades that followed (Collins et al., 2011; Marlatt, 1996). Nonetheless, this groundbreaking research in controlled drinking opened the door for a host of efficacious and more client-centered *moderate drinking* interventions for at-risk drinkers in the 1980s and 1990s (Sobell & Sobell, 1995).

1.5.2 Brief Interventions in Health Care Settings

With their way paved by the aforementioned early work in controlled drinking, brief and often opportunistic interventions for at-risk drinkers (e.g., clients in the emergency department) emerged as a strong approach to secondary prevention. In various meta-analyses, brief interventions in health care settings that featured either abstinence-based or moderate-drinking messaging showed modest efficacy (Angus et al., 2014; O'Donnell et al., 2013). It should, however, be noted that some researchers have questioned the strength of these effects (McCambridge & Saitz, 2017).

While most brief interventions have focused on promoting drinking reduction or abstinence, one of these interventions, the Brief Alcohol Screening Intervention for College Students (BASICS), marked the introduction of more clearly harm reduction–oriented strategies into brief interventions for at-risk drinkers (Dimeff et al., 1999). For this nondisordered, "risky drinking," college student population, BASICS has been shown to be efficacious in reducing both alcohol use and alcohol-related harm (Fachini et al., 2012).

1.5.3 Personalized Normative Feedback Interventions

Personalized normative feedback pairs information about one's drinking with peer norms, often in narrative and visual formats, to help people develop a sense of a discrepancy between their current drinking and that of their peers. Originally a component of larger, in-person interventions (e.g., BASICS, motivational enhancement therapy; SAMHSA, 1999), personalized normative feedback was later isolated as a stand-alone intervention via mailed or Web-based information (Larimer & Cronce, 2007). Occasionally, personalized normative feedback has explicitly included feedback on the recipients' alcohol-related harm (e.g., Collins et al., 2002) or harm reduction information (e.g., protective behavioral strategies), which has shown mixed effects in association with alcohol outcomes in nondisordered, at-risk drinking populations (Pearson, 2013).

1.5.4 Motivational Interviewing

Motivational interviewing is a person-centered psychotherapeutic approach for people who use substances (Rogers, 1957; Miller & Rollnick, 2013). In motivational interviewing, clinicians guide clients through examination of their ambivalence about their substance use, engaging active listening (i.e., open-ended questions, affirmations, reflections, and summary statements). Ultimately, the clinician should guide clients through their own development of discrepancy between their current use and desired outcomes and the resolution of that discrepancy in the direction of positive behavior change. Key to this approach is the motivational interviewing "spirit" which emphasizes partnership, acceptance, compassion, and evocation of clients' own motivation for change. Motivational interviewing also comprises sequential processes of clinical intervention, including engaging clients, focusing in on specific treatment goals, evoking motivation for change, and planning to systematically work toward goals. Motivational interviewing goals typically focus on "reducing substance use and related suffering" (Miller & Rollnick, 2013). Initially developed to help clients commit to abstinence-based treatment attendance (Miller, 1996), motivational interviewing has subsequently been recognized through research as an effective stand-alone and low-intensity way to help people with SUD achieve abstinence. More recently, it has been successfully used to encourage reduced use in nondisordered populations. In the Chapter 4 section "Engaging in Active Listening Throughout HaRT Sessions" we show how to apply motivational interviewing principles within harm reduction treatment.

1.5.5 Guided Self-Change

Primarily intended for nonclinical or less severely impacted populations (e.g., "problem drinkers" and what is now referred to in the DSM-5 as mild to moderate SUD diagnosis), *guided self-change* was developed in the early 1980s and refined throughout the 1990s and early 2000s by Sobell and Sobell (2005) and their colleagues. Guided self-change integrates cognitive-behavioral, motivational interviewing, and stepped-care principles, and has been packaged into one-on-one interventions, group sessions, mailed feedback interventions, and bibliotherapy. Defining elements include motivational interviewing style, provision of personalized feedback, readings and homework (e.g., decisional balance), self-monitoring of substance use, client selection of goals (with the exception of clients mandated to treatment), and cognitive aspects of relapse prevention. L. C. Sobell (personal communication, November 2, 2021) has indicated that most individuals with nonsevere AUD in guided self-change will seek to reduce rather than stop drinking, and thus, the most appropriate endpoint to evaluate its efficacy is drinking reduction or "low-risk drinking" (i.e., National Institute on Alcohol Abuse and Alcoholism criteria of < 4 drinks per day and < 8 per week for women; < 5 drinks per day and < 15 per week for men). In guided self-change studies, these data have been gathered using the *timeline followback method*. Days considered successful could involve abstinence or "low-risk drinking." For treatment of other SUDs, where any use was illegal according to the law at the time that work was conducted, the main outcome variable was days of abstinence.

While findings have been mixed and the specific components and modalities under the guided self-change umbrella have varied across time (Tucker & Simpson, 2011), the underlying principle that people can make changes on their own and that clinicians should strive to support client-desired change has provided an inspiration for harm reduction treatments and interventions that have followed.

1.5.6 Harm Reduction Psychotherapy

Starting in the early 2000s, psychologists in clinical practice who were frustrated with the punitive measures they observed in abstinence-based substance use treatment settings forged a new pathway: *harm reduction psychotherapy* (Denning & Little, 2012; Tartarsky, 2002). Harm reduction psychotherapy is more closely affiliated with the harm reduction movement and its tenets than the aforementioned evidence-based practices from the alcohol research field (see Sections 1.5.1 through 1.5.5). Although not empirically tested, harm reduction psychotherapies integrate various empirically established psychotherapeutic orientations and practices, including psychodynamic psychotherapy, motivational interviewing, and cognitive-behavioral approaches, toward a harm reduction end.

Self-help books for harm reduction have also proliferated, and two of these are more firmly rooted in the larger harm reduction movement (Anderson, 2010; Denning & Little, 2017). One of these authors, Kenneth Anderson, MA, a long-time harm reductionist with lived experience of homelessness and AUD, also created the Harm Reduction, Abstinence and Moderation Support (HAMS) website (https://hams.cc/), which provides harm reduction information, a podcast, an online support forum, chat room, email group, social media group, and live meetings. The aim is to help people choose their own goals around safer drinking, reduced drinking, or abstinence.

Although harm reduction psychotherapy and these related approaches are not evidence-based per se, their positive influence in the field is immeasurable, and this work has paved the way for us as clinicians and researchers as well. Communication and collaboration between researchers and harm reduction clinicians is on the rise, as are evaluation efforts. For example, a recent cross-sectional study asked 57 HAMS website users to retrospectively compare their alcohol outcomes before and after use of the website (Haug et al., 2020). Participants estimated they were consuming less alcohol subsequent to their use of the website, with those more engaged across website activities reporting greater reductions.

1.6 Conclusions

Harm reduction refers to a larger set of strategies that can be administered at the individual, community, population, and policy levels to help people who use substances, their families, and their communities reduce substance-related harm and improve QoL. In this book, we are focusing on the individual-level application of harm reduction in providing harm reduction treatment, or HaRT, for people who use substances. While we are introducing a new evidence-based practice, we acknowledge the vital foundational work done by our colleagues in substance use research and in the harm reduction movement that has informed the development of HaRT and shaped the larger substance use treatment landscape. Building on this foundation, we conducted 15 years of community-based participatory research during which we cocreated HaRT, together with people who use substances and the community-based agencies that serve them. Our collective vision was to destigmatize substance use and substance use treatment, contribute in a positive way to the social justice efforts of the larger harm reduction movement, and better fulfill community members' own vision for optimal healing and recovery pathways. The resulting HaRT bears a pragmatic mindset and compassionate heartset. Within that framework, harm reduction clinicians administer three primary treatment components: client-led measurement and tracking of harm reduction metrics, elicitation of clients' harm reduction and QoL goals and progress made toward them, and discussion of safer-use strategies and relative risks.

2

Theories and Models

The research literature is teeming with meta-analyses and systematic reviews of policy, population-based, and community-level harm reduction approaches. On the individual level, which is where most psychotherapists and counselors are focusing their work, a strong evidence base has documented the efficacy and effectiveness of pharmacological treatment to support harm reduction and even training in the provision of medication for opioid use disorder, more specifically (Cooper et al., 2020; Ma et al., 2019; Maglione et al., 2018). Until very recently, however, there have been very few evidence-based medication management or behavioral approaches to harm reduction treatment for SUD that could bolster the effects of harm reduction medications or serve as stand-alone interventions.

In this chapter, we will review models and theories undergirding harm reduction and HaRT, more specifically. First, we will review pharmacological treatments supporting harm reduction. Second, we will introduce the HaRT model and its theoretical and empirical underpinnings. At the end of the chapter, additional well-established but non-evidence-based approaches to harm reduction (Section 2.3: What HaRT Is *Not*) will be briefly reviewed for additional context.

2.1 Pharmacological Treatment for Harm Reduction

The development of pharmacological treatments that support harm reduction has been less informed by a unified theory and more informed by serendipitous discoveries and pragmatic yet somewhat siloed efforts to address pressing clinical needs.

> Best practices include naloxone for overdose reversal and opioid agonists to treat OUD

In the context of treatment for opioid use disorder (OUD), methadone and buprenorphine/naloxone, which are pharmaceutical grade controlled-dose opioid agonists, have become the clinical gold standards. Both are effective in reducing relapse to illicit opioids (Tkacz et al., 2012), and when taken regularly and over a long period of time, in preventing overdose-related mortality (Ma et al., 2019). Naloxone, an opioid antagonist also known as the overdose rescue drug, is effective in reversing overdose and saving lives (Chimbar & Moleta, 2018). For the first 4 decades after it was developed in 1961, naloxone was primarily available to medical professionals, with some lay distribution through needle and syringe exchange programs. Over the past 20 years, however, naloxone has become increasingly available to laypeople. Naloxone is now nationally and internationally recognized as a key means of saving lives in the opioid epidemic.

For AUD, naltrexone, an opioid antagonist available in extended-release injectable and oral formulations, and acamprosate, an oral medication believed to act on the glutaminergic system, have garnered the strongest and most consistent treatment outcomes to date (Ray et al., 2019). Supporting their ability to be integrated into harm reduction treatment, both naltrexone and acamprosate are safe for people who drink alcohol and have been shown to help people reduce heavy drinking episodes (Ray et al., 2019). The effectiveness of pharmacological treatment for other SUDs to date has been weaker and less consistent (Collins, Duncan, et al., 2016).

>**Naltrexone and acamprosate have the strongest and most consistent treatment effects for AUD**

This nearly exclusive focus on the evaluation of pharmacological treatment for individual-level harm reduction has been important to establish these treatments as helpful adjuncts for clients' harm reduction efforts. At the same time, there is a new emphasis in the terminology shift from "medication-assisted treatment" to "medication for opioid use disorder" that medication *is* the primary treatment (Winograd et al., 2019). Although well-intended, in that physicians want to ensure speedy access to life-saving medications, this move inadvertently eclipses the development of parallel behavioral treatment or counseling approaches for harm reduction that can be used as an adjunct to pharmacotherapy.

There follows an additional question: If medication is such an effective treatment approach that clients do not need behavioral treatment, why not just give clients medication without any conversation at all? The evidence-based response is that medication is effective only if clients are engaged and retained in treatment. The reality is that engagement and retention in medication-assisted treatment is relatively low, especially in more marginalized communities (Timko et al., 2016). We also know that treatment effects are bolstered by a strong therapeutic bond conveyed through clinicians' conversations with clients during what is often termed "medication management."

>**Although medications to support harm reduction are effective, they often have low levels of adherence**

The challenge is that all evidence-based medication management created to run alongside these pharmacological adjuncts has been focused on abstinence achievement instead of harm reduction. Thus, when clients do talk to clinicians about their substance use, there is often a disconnect between (a) the medication's function to reduce harm and (b) the clinician's advice to quit. This disconnect can be confusing for clients and clinicians alike. For example, clients have told us they do not understand why they are, on the one hand, being prescribed an opioid (e.g., methadone), and on the other hand, told they need to be abstinent from opioids. For their part, clinicians often set arbitrary rules in their programs that are often well-intended, but unnecessary and even counterproductive from a harm reduction perspective (e.g., ejecting clients from medication-assisted treatment program for opioids if they report using other substances).

Ultimately, this is where behavioral approaches, including briefer harm reduction medication management and longer-format harm reduction treatment, can be helpful. Regardless of our professional identities (e.g., physician, nurse, psychologist, case manager, social worker), we can equip ourselves with the knowledge to better understand individual clients' relative risks, talk to clients about staying safer and healthier when they use sub-

>**Pairing behavioral and pharmacological treatments can boost harm reduction benefit**

stances, and better support them in achieving their own harm reduction and QoL goals. This idea now has empirical support: A recent study conducted by our team has shown that combining behavioral and pharmacological harm reduction approaches can synergistically boost the impact of both, improving engagement and efficacy (Collins, Duncan, et al., 2021).

In the next section, we will talk about HaRT as a behavioral or psychotherapeutic way to engage clients – be it in medication management or in counseling alone – that parallels the purpose of the medications our clients are being prescribed.

2.2 Behavioral Harm Reduction Treatment

HaRT primarily entails brief counseling that aims to meet people "where they're at" both in their motivation for change and in their communities. It is inherently flexible because it requires neither an abstinence-based treatment goal nor an abstinence-based treatment setting. It assumes the same ecological systems framework discussed in prior sections, which holds that substance use is not only influenced by individual-level factors, but also broader familial, community, social, economic, and even geopolitical factors (Bronfenbrenner, 1979). Because SUD is not viewed as residing solely within the individual, harm reduction clinicians avoid pathologizing or placing moral value on substance use (Denning & Little, 2012). Instead, they provide community members with the information they need to make scientifically and clinically informed – but personally made – decisions to reduce their substance-related harm and improve their QoL for themselves, their families, and their communities.

There has been some disagreement about what differentiates a harm reduction approach from other treatment approaches (Heather, 2006). It is, however, the primary therapeutic intention – *harm reduction* versus *use reduction* or abstinence – that provides the clearest point of differentiation (Collins et al., 2011; Heather, 2006). Additionally, the therapeutic intention of HaRT is transparent and explicit, whereas abstinence or use reduction treatment goals are often assumed or implied in most other approaches.

Abstinence has long served as the required focus of nearly all substance use treatment services available in the US. Just this year, however, harm reduction has garnered policy support from the White House, Executive Office of the President, and the Office of National Drug Control Policy (2022), with federal agencies announcing expanded definitions of recovery to include non-abstinence-based outcomes (Hagman et al., 2022). Researchers have also long noted the need for harm reduction treatment approaches (e.g., Marlatt & Witkiewitz, 2002), and the importance of honoring client-directed change (e.g., Sobell et al., 2000). Indeed, behavioral harm reduction interventions have garnered an evidence base for minimizing alcohol-related harm in nonclinical populations (e.g., college drinkers; Fachini et al., 2012; Pearson, 2013). Additionally, work has been done, particularly in alcohol research and treatment, to begin to broaden the definition of recovery (Witkiewitz et al., 2021; Witkiewitz et al., 2020). Finally, colleagues in the harm reduction field have developed psychotherapeutic practices, clinician manuals, and self-help guides (e.g., Anderson, 2010; Denning & Little, 2012, 2017; Tartarsky, 2002). Thus, the tradition of individual-level harm reduction approaches and the acknowledgment of the need for individual-level harm reduction approaches for SUD is not new.

HaRT builds on this growing interest in harm reduction and client-led approaches. In Section 1.4 we outline the HaRT model (see Figure 1) and its theoretical underpinnings in more detail.

2.2.1 HaRT Mindset

The *HaRT mindset* supports the realization of client-driven goals and recognizes any client-led movement toward reducing harm and improving QoL as positive steps in recovery (Marlatt, 1998a). It is important to reiterate that "recovery" in harm reduction does not automatically imply abstinence, moderation, or use reduction, or compliance with clinicians' conceptualization of recovery. In Table 1 and in the following section, we delineate the assumptions that are inherent in the use reduction mindset (wherein the "doctor knows best") and the harm reduction mindset, wherein we support client-driven goal setting because the "client knows better."

> The HaRT mindset is transparent, pragmatic and focuses on a mutual understanding of clients' relative risks and safety

Table 1
Illustrating the Differences Between the Use Reduction and Harm Reduction Mindsets

Use reduction	Harm reduction
• Ultimate goal is abstinence.	• Ultimate goal is harm reduction.
• Use and harm correlate 1:1.	• Use and harm do not correlate 1:1.
• Role is prescriptive: Clinician "prescribes" treatment goal and pathway.	• Role is predictive: Clinician helps client assess their risk for harm and develop ways to reduce risk.
• Doctor knows best!	• Client knows better!

Harm Reduction Is the Ultimate Goal

There are important reasons for the prioritization of client-driven, harm reduction goals over provider-driven, use reduction goals. First, the focus on harm reduction versus use reduction is pragmatic. We acknowledge that life-long abstinence is one viable means of reducing substance-related harm, and abstinence-based treatment presents one viable pathway to that end. However, the vast majority of people who use substances – even those with SUD – are not ready, willing, or able to stop using or attend abstinence-based treatment (SAMHSA, 2022). Thus, client-driven and harm reduction pathways are more intrinsically appealing, lower barrier, and more inclusive of the broader spectrum of people with SUD. This positions harm reduction goals as more engaging and harm reduction treatment as having greater reach than the de facto narrower focus on abstinence-based goals via abstinence-based

> HaRT expands our reach to clients who are not ready, willing, or able to attend abstinence-based treatment

treatment (see Box 3 for community perspectives on the appealing nature of harm reduction, especially for marginalized populations).

> **Box 3**
> **Community Advisory Board Member, Grover "Will" Williams, On Why We Prioritize Harm Reduction Over Use Reduction (Collins et al., 2022)**
>
> "If one is motivated – self-motivated, perhaps by having 'hit bottom' – abstinence is possible under the ideal circumstances. However, many in the homeless community are not living under ideal circumstances. It's not the option of abstinence that does more harm than good, it's the requirement that makes it more difficult and unrealistic. ... Harm reduction, with its less rigid structure, allows for some flexibility. This seems appropriate in cases where, due to chaotic circumstances such as homelessness, people have less ability to keep to a strictly defined routine. It can help fill the gap. It's about progress, not perfection."

Substance Use and Substance-Related Harm Are Not Correlated 1:1
Abstinence-based approaches are predicated on the belief, embraced by various schools of thought ranging from Alcoholics Anonymous to the stepped-care model, that the more one uses substances, the more substance-related harm one experiences. The corollary is that the more one reduces use and ultimately achieves abstinence, the more one's substance-related harm will decrease. However, this assumed one-to-one correlation between use reduction and harm reduction does not consistently hold. As noted in Chapter 1, research conducted around the world has consistently shown that larger familial, community-wide, and even geopolitical forces create disparities that precipitate and maintain a disproportionate level of substance-related harm in more marginalized and vulnerable populations, even after controlling for the amount of use (Collins, 2016). Such higher-level, systemic factors can interact with individual-level, biological factors to further complicate this assumed one-to-one correlation between use reduction and harm reduction (to see how this plays out, see Box 4).

Because the assumed one-to-one relationship between the spectrum of substance use and the spectrum of substance-related harm does not hold, particularly in marginalized communities (Collins, 2016), harm reduction clinicians apply Occam's razor or the law of parsimony. We relinquish our need to force the spectrum of substance use to align with the spectrum of substance-related harm, and we simply focus on the latter. As a corollary, we release the system's pressure on us to force use reduction and abstinence as the sole solution for reducing our clients' experience of substance-related harm. Again, we simply focus on the latter. When we do so, we are freed to focus on the most relevant, straightforward, effective, and pragmatic means for the individual, their families, and their communities to reduce substance-related harm and improve QoL. We open ourselves to attending to our clients' own needs and goals, and more local community-based means of achieving them. We open ourselves to, in the words of the Chicago Recovery Alliance, the power of "any positive change."

When freed from trying to align the spectra of use and harm, clients can focus on reducing substance-related harm

> **Box 4**
> **How Can Well-Intentioned Abstinence-Based Systems End Up Perpetuating Substance-Related Harm?**
>
> The criminalization of public intoxication (systemic factor) disproportionately impacts people experiencing homelessness and AUD, who have no private space to consume alcohol (systemic factor). The resulting cycles of heavy alcohol use due to AUD (individual-level factor) and involuntary abstinence due to incarceration and mandated treatment spurred by public intoxication charges (systemic factor) can precipitate the kindling effect (individual-level factor), which results in increasingly severe and potentially deadly withdrawal symptoms with each return to abstinence (Becker, 1998). Thus, for those who are physiologically dependent and not ready, willing, or able to achieve abstinence, *drinking some alcohol every day and thereby avoiding withdrawal and its kindling effect can be less harmful than circling the revolving door of jail and treatment.* This is a known medical phenomenon, and there have been grassroots efforts to educate community members on harm reduction to address it. Nonetheless, our existing treatment systems do not recognize or allow for clients to use alcohol to "get well" or avoid withdrawal, and self-led or medically assisted alcohol tapers are not considered viable options by treatment providers.

Role of Harm Reduction Clinicians Is Predictive, Not Prescriptive

The overarching aim of HaRT is to help people who use substances, their families, and their communities reduce substance-related harm and improve QoL. It is, however, also emphasized that these aims are broadly conceived, so clients can define their own recovery pathway. Clients may invite harm reduction clinicians to walk with them along their recovery pathways, and the two parties engage in co-learning about the relative risks of substance use in the clients' life context. Clients have their own specialized knowledge around the drug (quantity, frequency, harm, modes of use), set (motivational, emotional), and setting (environment, other people involved) that they can share with the clinician, and the clinician has access to specialized knowledge in ways to alter or work within the drug, set, and setting to reduce the relative risks involved (Denning & Little, 2012). Thus, when the client arrives at a fork in the path, harm reduction clinicians may share specialized knowledge (i.e., information about safer use, relative risks) to empower clients to make even more scientifically informed decisions about their substance use moving forward.

Harm reduction clinicians empower clients with information about relative risks

2.2.2 HaRT Heartset

The heartset entails a culturally humble, compassionate way of being with a client. In this case, compassion refers to "feeling with" the client, coupled with an unconflicted desire to remove suffering and to support client-defined and client-led treatment goals, intentions, prayers, or hopes. This compassionate way of being is conveyed through means that will be familiar to those who practice motivational interviewing: openness to, acceptance of, and

The HaRT heartset entails cultural humility, compassion, acceptance, and advocacy

fundamental respect for the shared humanity with the *other* and the other's values, beliefs, concerns, and priorities (Miller & Rollnick, 2013).

HaRT then builds further upon these client-centered values by supporting clients in setting, striving toward, and achieving exclusively client-led goals, providing the opportunity for transformative change through intrinsic rather than extrinsic motivation. Clinicians balance this support with complete transparency regarding their role in the system and its limitations (e.g., acknowledging the oppressive nature of the systems clients must navigate, including our own research and treatment institutions) and the harm reduction agenda (i.e., harm reduction and QoL improvement).

Finally, clinicians engage in advocacy for clients and help clients advocate for themselves. For example, clinicians may facilitate connections to needed and desired harm reduction (e.g., needle and syringe exchange) and other social services (e.g., housing and legal advocates), might accompany clients to appointments to bear witness to their treatment or gently educate other providers, and introduce clients to community-based harm reduction agencies to engage in community advocacy. The mindset and heartset are conveyed to clients at the beginning of HaRT, and throughout the sessions, to remain transparent about the harm reduction clinician's role and to remind clients of the rationale for the treatment they are cocreating with clinicians.

2.2.3 HaRT Components

Tracking client-preferred recovery metrics, harm-reduction goal-setting, and safer-use strategies

The three HaRT components are delivered in the context of the mindset and heartset and include (a) collaborative assessment and tracking of client-preferred substance use metrics, (b) elicitation of clients' harm reduction and QoL goals, and (c) discussion of safer-use strategies. These three components are detailed in a step-by-step guide in Chapter 4.

Collaborative Assessment and Tracking of Client-Preferred Substance Use Metrics

For the first component, clinicians work with clients to holistically assess and track over time relevant substance use, substance-related harm, and other client-prioritized metrics (see Section 3.3.2 for measures of outcomes). Clinicians help clients create a graphic representation of their progress, which is updated monthly (see Figure 14 and Figure 15). Clinicians elicit clients' narratives around their trajectories across key metrics and affirm positive changes. In the case of flat or worsening trajectories, clinicians provide affirmation for other efforts toward healing (e.g., attendance at HaRT sessions), encouragement for clients to continue their efforts moving forward, and troubleshooting to improve the helpfulness of HaRT to the client. See Chapter 4 for step-by-step instructions on this process.

Elicitation of Clients' Harm Reduction and QoL Goals

For the second component, clinicians elicit clients' harm reduction and QoL goals and assess progress made toward them. As a reminder, HaRT does not assume abstinence or use reduction goals; thus, we clinicians are open to whatever goals clients believe can reduce their substance-related harm and improve their QoL. We start our discussion about harm reduction goals by asking clients, "What do you want to see happen for yourself?" This is a simple but transformative question for many clients in substance use treatment (see Box 5).

> **Box 5**
> **Joey Stanton, Community Consultant, On the Importance of Client-Led Harm Reduction Goal Setting (Collins, Black Bear, et al., 2018)**
>
> "I am amazed at what my life has become now. I have a job. I have a relationship with my daughter! I am leaving for New Orleans for a month to be with my grandson. Oh my god! I not gonna say none of this would have happened without Susan and Seema because that would be bullshit. What happened was that people started talking to me like a human being. People started talking to me, asking me what I wanted. What my goals were."

As a means of preparing ourselves for this new diversity of goal setting in substance use treatment, our research team has conducted a series of mixed methods studies to ascertain the content of goals generated in the HaRT context (Collins, Grazioli, et al., 2015; Fentress et al., 2021). A breakdown of these client-generated, initial treatment goals is shown in Figure 3.

As indicated in Figure 3, 28% of client-driven goals were substance-related. Of note, only 5% of client-stated goals entailed abstinence achievement; other substance-related goals included reducing use, reducing substance-related harm, decreasing contact with triggers, and connecting with recovery supports. Clients also expressed interest in meeting their basic needs (25%; including obtaining housing, accessing services), attaining greater QoL (24%; engaging in meaningful activities, reconnecting with meaningful relationships), improving physical and mental health outcomes (16%), and other assorted goals, including improved money management, activities of daily living, and personal safety (7%).

Clinicians record clients' weekly harm reduction goals and collaboratively assess at subsequent sessions whether clients have fully, partially, or not achieved their stated goals. Clinicians use a sense of curiosity and wonder by way of open-ended questions and strengths-based reflections to elicit clients' stories about their progress toward their harm reduction goals and provide affirmations and encouragement to support ongoing goal actualization. Regardless of clients' progress toward their goals, clinicians remain supportive and accepting of clients and offer reflections and affirmations of efforts and inherent strengths (e.g., "It didn't work out exactly as planned. But you know what? You showed up today to keep working at it, and that's pretty rad.") Clinicians also help clients break down goals into smaller, more achievable stepwise goals, and engage in troubleshooting to help remove barriers to their realization. The point of harm reduction goal setting is not to prioritize clinicians' goals but to build clients' sense of self-efficacy and autonomy in creating, striving toward, and achieving their own goals from week to week.

Our research with marginalized people with SUD indicates only a small minority want abstinence

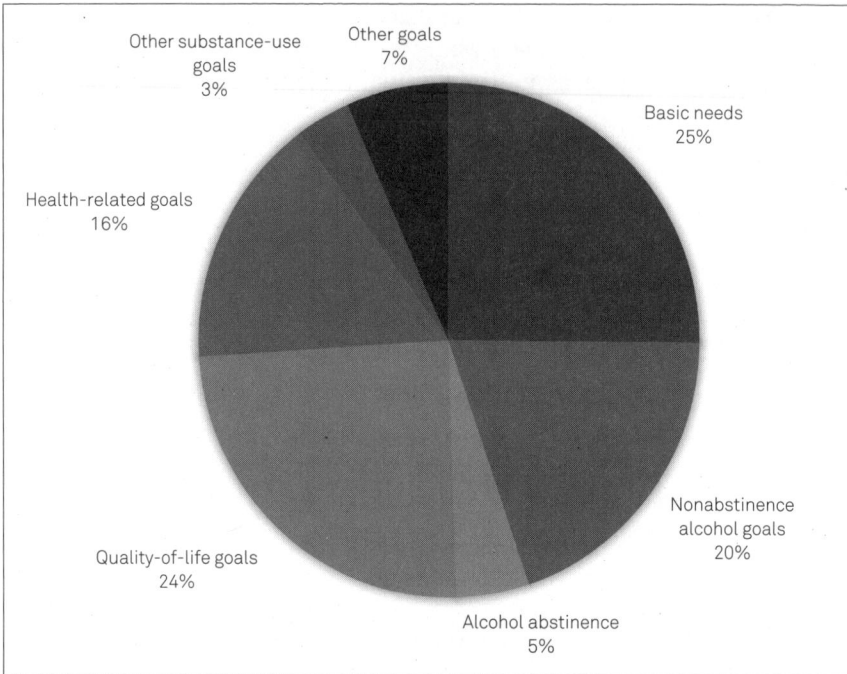

Figure 3
Stated harm reduction goals among non-treatment-seeking people experiencing homelessness, alcohol use disorder, and/or polysubstance use (N = 325). Of particular note, only 5% of stated goals entail achieving alcohol abstinence, in a population severely affected by alcohol use disorder. Based on Fentress et al., 2021.

Discussion of Safer-Use Strategies

Safer-use strategies are ways to stay healthier when using, change the manner of use for safety, and reduce use

The third component entails discussion of the relative risks and benefits of clients' current substance use and strategies that can help them (a) stay healthier when using (e.g., drinking water to stay hydrated, taking B-complex vitamins to avoid thiamine deficiency in the context of heavy alcohol use), (b) alter the manner in which they use to be safer (e.g., not mixing drugs and alcohol, ensuring they do not use alone in the case of opioid overdose), or (c) change the amount they use (e.g., use reduction, abstinence). If reduction or abstinence is a goal, and a client is physiologically dependent on alcohol or benzodiazepines, interventionists review information on the risks of withdrawal as well as self-tapering schedules (Anderson, 2010), or the possibility of a medically supervised withdrawal. In the case of opioids, this discussion might be around referrals for medication for opioid use disorder to manage withdrawal and relapse and overdose risk. This discussion is facilitated by safer-use handouts that give clients information to make more scientifically informed decisions about their use (see sample in Figure 13 and Appendix 1 for handouts).

Pharmacological Support

A fourth component – pharmacological adjuncts and medication-assisted treatment, such as those discussed earlier in this chapter, in Section 2.1 – can be added to further bolster clients' harm reduction outcomes, goals, and safer-use strategies. Evidence-based pharmacological adjuncts that support harm reduction include naloxone to reverse opioid overdose; buprenorphine and methadone to stave off withdrawal, decrease overdose risk, and as relevant, prevent relapse to illicit opioids; naltrexone and acamprosate for AUD; and safer nicotine products (ranging from smokeless tobacco, to electronic nicotine delivery systems, to nicotine replacement therapy).

> The behavioral aspects of HaRT can be combined with pharmacological support to boost treatment effectiveness

2.3 What HaRT Is *Not*

We deeply appreciate the assertion made in other practices that defining what a construct *is not* is just as important as defining what it *is* (Miller & Rollnick, 2009). In this case, defining what HaRT *is not* serves a specific purpose. We do not wish to minimize the importance of other evidence-based approaches to substance use intervention and treatment (e.g., cognitive behavior treatment, relapse prevention, 12-step facilitation, motivational interviewing, mindfulness-based relapse prevention, and contingency management), but rather to circumscribe what is unique to HaRT so providers can more confidently engage in the practice and be transparent with clients about their treatment rationale and planning.

Because this question often comes up in trainings and in conversation with other researchers and clinicians, we created the slide featured in Figure 4.

In fact, what all the evidence-based treatment modalities listed in Figure 4 share is the underlying assumption that the clinician (or researcher) knows best and that, when there is disagreement – even subtle, unspoken, or unknown to one of the parties – about appropriate goals (i.e., abstinence or

> HaRT was codeveloped with community members and prioritizes their perspectives and goals

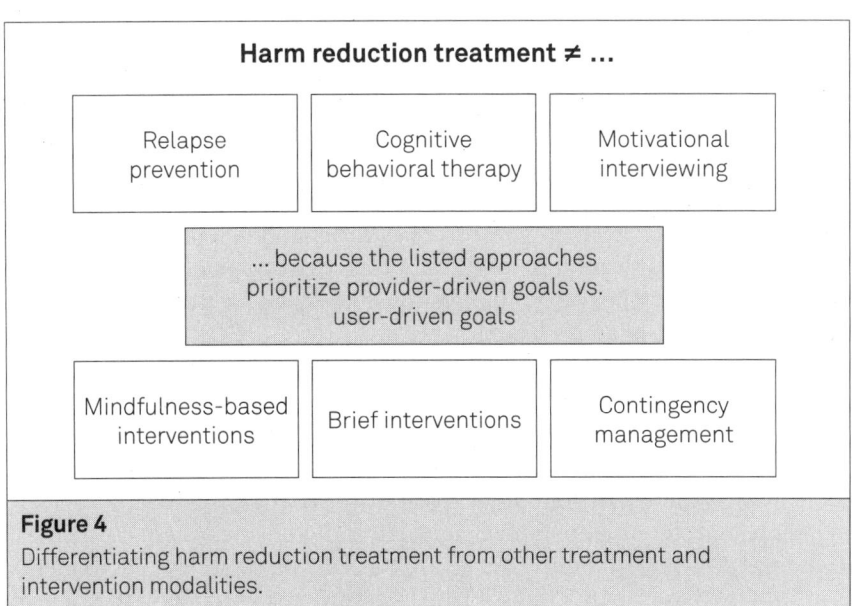

Figure 4
Differentiating harm reduction treatment from other treatment and intervention modalities.

use reduction) and optimal treatment course (stepped care; participation in the treatment system), the clinician's perspective may take precedence over the clients'. This fact is often not even up to the clinician; it is so seamlessly integrated into our treatment systems that, ultimately, the doctor knows best. Clients are then guided toward these provider-driven goals and treatment pathways. Different substance use treatment approaches often utilize different strategies to engage and align people with provider-driven goals, which often entail abstinence and/or abstinence-based treatment attendance (see Box 6).

> **Box 6**
> **How the Use-Reduction and Abstinence-Based Mindset Has Been Embedded in Substance Use Treatment and Conveyed to Clients**
>
> One approach has been to both explicitly state and simultaneously assume clients' acquiescence with use reduction or abstinence-based goals (e.g., relapse prevention; Marlatt & Gordon, 1985). Other pathways more subtly assume provider-endorsed and use-reduction and abstinence-based goals and then seek to align clients with these goals using social and psychological principles. For example, behavioral approaches make use of classical conditioning (e.g., cue exposure, aversion therapy) and/or operant conditioning (e.g., contingency management, behavioral contracting). Other approaches additionally capitalize on social learning principles (e.g., CRAFT, 12-step facilitation, Johnson-style interventions). Motivational interviewing uses engagement, focusing, and evocation processes to guide the client in developing and resolving discrepancies in the direction of what the "counselor regards to be appropriate goals" (Miller & Rollnick, 2013).

In contrast, HaRT is less directive in its approach. While the name does convey its agenda, HaRT is highly flexible and thus can easily and must necessarily accommodate any client-driven goals that can reduce substance-related harm (e.g., reduced blackouts, avoiding withdrawal, abstinence) and/or improve QoL within a person's own context and community (Collins et al., 2015).

At this point in the training, an attendee will often ask, "But what about motivational interviewing, though? Isn't that harm reduction?" As part of the generation that grew up with motivational interviewing in our graduate and postdoctoral training, we embrace the compassionate motivational interviewing style or spirit which now serves as a foundational means of engagement and communication across many treatment approaches. In fact, in Chapter 4, we draw heavily on motivational interviewing's emphasis on and operationalization of active listening skills.

Motivational interviewing is, however, not synonymous with harm reduction, or HaRT, more specifically. As Miller noted in our personal communication, HaRT shares the compassionate spirit of motivational interviewing but within the context of harm reduction goal setting and psychoeducation (W. R. Miller, personal communication, May 15, 2018). Indeed, the clearest points of differentiation between HaRT and other treatment modalities, including motivational interviewing, are the specific treatment components that form the basis of HaRT sessions – assessing harm reduction metrics for collaborative tracking, eliciting harm reduction goals, and discussing safer-use strategies – which are not found in the aforementioned substance use treatment modalities.

More abstractly, there is a larger underlying and philosophical difference. Even in the most recent edition of *Motivational Interviewing: Helping People Change*, Chapter 10 is titled "When Goals Differ," and Miller and Rollnick (2013) note that "therapists from a humanistic or existential orientation" – and one could insert harm reduction there – "might object to the directional aspect of motivational interviewing, whereby clients are intentionally guided towards what the counselor regards to be appropriate goals" (Miller & Rollnick, 2013). In contrast, in this book and in HaRT, you will find no "When Goals Differ" chapter, because the goals of a harm reduction clinician will never differ from those of their clients. We always center the clients' goals, setting aside what we "regard to be appropriate goals." In doing so, we decenter ourselves and our value set, and embrace the clients'.

That is not to say that we do not have any agenda as harm reduction clinicians. We offer freely and openly to clients that, as harm reduction clinicians, we aim to help people, families, and communities reduce their experience of substance-related harm and improve their QoL. However, we ensure we are transparent about the treatment rationale from the start, and after working with hundreds of clients and research participants, we have learned that everyone wants to see something positive happen for themselves, their families, and their communities. Largely, these client-driven goals are easy for us to endorse as clinically meaningful goals. The perk is that they are also coming from the client so automatically carry more weight and investment. Once we have all "unlearned" our institutionally driven bias toward abstinence, then client-driven, harm reduction goal setting becomes easier for the client because they do not have to figure out what we want to hear. It is also easier for us because we do not have to convince clients they need to embrace a certain recovery pathway or set of goals. Our research suggests this latter point saves us from experiencing the discord that arises in abstinence-based treatment *when goals differ*. Because we recognize the client knows best, we defer to the client, and we generally find that discord does not come up (Collins, Clifasefi, Dana, et al., 2012; Collins, Jones, et al., 2016).

Given the chance, clients generate clinically meaningful goals that we can support as clinicians

3

Assessment and Treatment Indications

3.1 Treatment Indication

To date, HaRT has been associated with reduced use and substance-related harm across three single-arm pilots (involving two alcohol trials and one smoking trial) and two randomized controlled trials (involving participants with AUD, with 80% of those with polysubstance use) in community-based settings and with hundreds of non-treatment-seeking individuals who were socially marginalized (i.e., experiencing or having lived experience of chronic homelessness; Collins, Clifasefi, et al., 2019; Collins, Duncan, et al., 2021; Collins, Nelson, et al., 2019). Since that time, we have implemented HaRT as an evidence-based treatment track at our institution and have used this treatment modality outside of the research context, observing clinically meaningful reductions in substance use and substance-related harm across clients with co-occurring psychiatric and SUD, including polysubstance use. Thus, both research and clinical experiences indicate HaRT can create clinically meaningful change across both non-treatment-seeking and outpatient treatment-seeking populations and across substances.

> Given its flexibility HaRT is indicated for most clients

In our research, only a small proportion of participants have expressed interest in abstinence-based goals at treatment intake (approximately 5%; Fentress et al., 2021; Grazioli et al., 2015); however, HaRT has worked well in engaging and treating clients who have a wide range of goals, from QoL goals, to safer-use goals to use reduction goals, to abstinence-based goals. This makes HaRT clinically convenient because of its flexible range. Of note, however, abstinence-based goals are congruent with HaRT only if they are strongly client-driven, well-founded, well-resourced, and falling clearly outside of the "premature focus trap" (i.e., clients and clinicians' tendency to want to move quickly toward abstinence without a strong motivational foundation or behavioral plan, often due to internalized shame about use, perceptions of clinician-preferred treatment goals, or systems pressures to stop using; Miller & Rollnick, 2013). Another clinically convenient feature is that other treatment modalities may be easily woven into HaRT, including motivational interviewing, cognitive-behavioral strategies, relapse prevention, and even 12-step facilitation for clients with abstinence-based goals who fully and voluntarily choose that ancillary support. Thus, HaRT provides a strong stand-alone treatment for both treatment-seekers and non-treatment seekers, across a wide range of goals, including but not limited to abstinence-based goals, and can be integrated with other evidence-based practices, as determined by clients' own interests and goals.

> Other interventions may be integrated into the flexible HaRT treatment course

3.2 Preparation for HaRT

In harm reduction, we acknowledge larger systems influences on our clients and our work; thus, this section serves as a continuation of the prior section's coverage of treatment indication. Specifically, this section will help you assess whether your practice *setting and system* are indicated for HaRT implementation, and if so, how to prepare yourself to navigate the system on your clients' behalf to ensure strong application of HaRT, which will be discussed in Chapter 4.

3.2.1 Reflecting On and Readying Your Practice Setting

Depending on the level of minoritization and marginalization of your client base, you might already be aware of your clients' experience of the systems in which we work. Here are a few examples of how we and our colleagues (too slowly) awakened to our role and complicity as clinicians and researchers in the interlocking systems of oppression. We noticed that people experiencing greater marginalization in our system (e.g., People of Color, LGBTQIA2+, womxn, people experiencing homelessness or houselessness, rural clients, clients experiencing more severe levels of substance-related harm, clients with co-occurring disorders) were often and variously subject to greater monitoring, offered fewer services, exposed to harsher treatment and service conditions, and/or experienced less flexibility and compassion from us and our settings. We realized a large proportion of substance use treatment serves *mandated clients* and often entails reporting to courts, probation or parole officers, or child protective services about clients' treatment attendance, self-reported substance use, and urine toxicology reports. We became increasingly concerned that our clients might be reincarcerated or lose custody of children based on reports we crafted. We noticed our own discomfort in our staffing meetings or in consultations in which clients and their lives were reduced to reporting on their level of use or experience of substance-related harm. Worse, we regretted conversations about our clients that dehumanized or belittled them (e.g., laughing, scoffing or rolling our eyes at their histories, experiences of relapse, behavior exhibited while intoxicated, or feeling they "had it coming" when they experienced substance-related harm).

Once we realized the harmful nature of our systems and our actions within them, we tried to find new ways forward by asking community members what *their* experience of our systems and our services had been. We learned across several studies that community members who had been marginalized in the system appreciated talking to counselors and clinicians about their physical and mental health and even about their substance use. However, they did not appreciate and reported shutting down when those conversations ended with overtures about abstinence, resulted in clinician-driven treatment plans and goals, and were shared – sometimes perceived as surreptitiously – with other entities (Collins, Clifasefi, Dana, et al., 2012; Collins, Jones, et al., 2016; Nelson et al., 2022).

When we asked people how they would redesign treatment in their own vision, they told us that intrinsically derived motivation and recovery pathways, *not* extrinsic pressures (e.g., mandated treatment), were associated with engagement and positive outcomes (Clifasefi et al., 2016; Collins, Jones, et al., 2016; Nelson et al., 2022). This insight corroborated our quantitative findings, which showed that intrinsic motivation for change and *not* the external pressures of treatment attendance was associated with changes in alcohol use and alcohol-related harm over time (Collins, Malone, et al., 2012). They preferred compassionate counselors with lived experience who could provide insights into recovery; they largely did not appreciate a "tough love" approach, institutional settings, or power struggles with counselors (Collins, Jones, et al., 2016; Nelson et al., 2022). They wanted more clinicians from their communities represented and more client-led and culturally aligned approaches (Clifasefi et al., 2016; Collins, Jones, et al., 2016; Nelson et al., 2022). They wanted help meeting their own goals, which often included substance-related goals, but just as often centered on meeting basic needs, reconnection with meaningful activities and relationships, and improving overall health and well-being (Collins, Grazioli, et al., 2015; Fentress et al., 2021).

These community observations and then construction of interventions and treatments following from these client-led principles formed the basis for the HaRT outlined in this chapter, which we first codeveloped and tested in research trials (Collins, Clifasefi, et al., 2019; Collins, Duncan, et al., 2021; Collins, Duncan, et al., 2015), and as recounted above, went on to implement in our university medical center.

However, we recognize that the population, the context, the specific settings, and the geographical location of our work over the past 15 years have strongly colored our perceptions of clients' interests. We also acknowledge that the specific spaces in which we work are often open to harm reduction and thus offer us more freedom to implement HaRT and incorporate clients' interests than other settings and locations might offer. One might be deeply ensconced in an abstinence-based treatment agency in a less progressive geographical location. Others on one's team may strongly hold the debunked

---

Box 7

What Do You Say If a Colleague Questions Your Use of a Harm Reduction Approach As "Enabling"?

Research has shown us that harm reduction approaches across the individual, community, and policy levels do *not* lead to increased use and harm. Contrary to the "enabling hypothesis," harm reduction approaches lead to decreased use and harm. HaRT specifically is associated with reduced substance use and substance-related harm across our various research studies. The research also shows us that:

1. Harm reduction helps you build better rapport and engagement. When people stay engaged, they stay alive.
2. When people commit to safer-use strategies, they experience decreases in substance-related harm.
3. People with drinking-related goals of any kind reduce their drinking and alcohol-related harm, and having more drinking and QoL goals leads to better health-related quality of life.

yet common belief that harm reduction work is "enabling" and may believe HaRT could be detrimental to clients (see Box 7 for evidence that debunks the incorrect yet widespread "enabling hypothesis"). One might be practicing in settings that are deeply networked with other agencies that require abstinence (e.g., housing, criminal justice). In our trainings, clinicians working in such settings often wonder aloud: Is it possible to practice HaRT or any harm reduction approaches with clients in such settings? How one can enact harm reduction when ensconced in these interlocking systems of oppression?

The answer is complex and depends on your professional role and the specific setting in which you are working. We have provided HaRT trainings for people working in criminal justice settings because we feel that more compassionate and pragmatic ways of working with people who use substances are always relevant. However, there are real concerns about "using" more compassionate means of communication and titles that obfuscate a person's role and can thus become coercive, disingenuous, and manipulative (see Box 8). This issue has surfaced and been addressed in other compassionate and more client-centered styles as well (Miller & Rollnick, 2013). However, it is even more crucial to address in the context of HaRT, which is a client-*driven* approach and should support and not belie the grassroots advocacy and activist movements that have long championed social justice and harm reduction in marginalized communities.

> **Box 8**
> **Aspiring Harm Reduction Clinicians Must Be Aware of Hidden Systems Exploitation**
>
> One concerning practice is the trend to rename probation officers "probation counselors." Defendants' confusion about the term "counselor" often inadvertently engenders a feeling of trust between probation or parole officers and defendants. Defendants then share more information, based on the implicit belief that "counselors" have ethical obligations to place clients' needs first and maintain client privacy and confidentiality. Instead, probation or parole officers are usually obliged to prioritize community and public safety, and they have no legal or ethical obligation to maintain defendants' confidentiality or privacy. So, when defendants feel they can share, for example, a relapse with their "counselor," they can find themselves additionally charged or reincarcerated due to a probation or parole violation. Our clients have reported feeling caught off-guard by this framing, and we have witnessed it firsthand. Clients' trust is violated, trauma retriggered, and personal freedom denied for being honest. We are not saying probation or parole officers intend for their positionality to play out in this way, but that is often how systemic oppression works.

HaRT requires client advocacy and absolute transparency about the practice and the systems in which we work. We all encounter systemic challenges and oppression, and we believe many of these barriers to practicing HaRT can be overcome with persistence, systems advocacy, and engagement, which we outline in the sections that follow. However, if this transparency and advocacy for clients is systemically impossible in your setting, we cannot condone calling it harm reduction, even as we are always happy to see

HaRT requires client advocacy and absolute transparency about the practice and the systems in which we work

people responding more compassionately and pragmatically to people who use substances.

Aside from these more extreme examples, we believe there are ways to practice HaRT responsibly, even given systems limitations. Key to fidelity to the model is understanding and defining your own positionality within the system, conveying your positionality to clients transparently and regularly, and advocating for harm reduction, more generally, and your clients, more specifically, within your system and other systems as well. We expound on how to enact these processes in the following sections.

3.2.2 Preparing to Navigate Systems For and With Clients

Once you have taken stock of the HaRT readiness of your setting and whether HaRT is a viable approach within it, you can make decisions about how you will navigate the system to better work for your clients as you implement HaRT in your practice. Here are some important steps.

Understanding and Defining Your Own Positionality in the System
It is important to understand what your setting can do for clients and what it cannot (e.g., treatment and other social service offerings), what its rules and norms are and how they are shaped (e.g., policies and procedures), and how you might be interfacing with other systems and entities (e.g., connection to funders and internal and external collaborators and agencies). Understand where *you are* in the larger organizational chart. How much referent, expert, and/or institutional power do you have to shape systems? How much can you define your own practice within the existing system? Consider these questions and your answers carefully. In section 4.1.1, we will discuss how to translate those to your clients through your treatment rationale and informed consent process.

Engaging in Systems-Level Advocacy

> Build and listen to community advisory boards; advocate to meet their stated needs; push back on dehumanizing practices

Even if you do not have a lot of institutional power, you can take steps to remedy problematic omissions or commissions in your own work and in your setting. First, consider where current practices do not align with the harm reduction principles discussed earlier in this book. Then, you may engage in the following numbered actions, as relevant for your setting and practice. Please note that these are suggested starting points and not an exhaustive list.
1. *Ensure that client and community voices are heard:* If possible, we recommend assembling a community advisory board of people with lived experience – the key stakeholders in, and individuals who represent end users of, your services – to inform the services you provide (for a research-based example of this process, see Collins, Clifasefi, et al., 2018). Be sure to compensate people for their time, provide refreshments, listen attentively, and include their suggestions liberally. If their suggestions do not align with existing services, rules or norms, or connections to other agencies, work on reshaping your services and systems to come into alignment with the community's expressed interests.

2. *Speak up where your setting might be omitting needed services:* With community input (when possible), inform management what services need to be added, reshaped, or removed to be maximally inclusive, equitable, healing, and acceptance-based for clients. We know from our own experience the fine balance between pushing the system successfully and getting oneself expulsed, and we recommend harm reduction clinicians walk that line carefully. If you are expulsed from the system, you cannot advocate for clients within it; however, it may be that socially just, harm reduction practices will not be supported in that environment, at least for now. If possible, you might choose to find a more amenable setting for this work.
3. *Push back against the systemic dehumanization of clients:* Reconsider waiting room protocols, systematic urine toxicology testing, and assessment styles that may initially and even inadvertently set up an adversarial tone or assertion of institutional power. Do not laugh at "gallows humor" in staffing meetings, and push back when dehumanizing stories are told about clients. Here is one strategy we adopted to curtail stigmatizing language in staffing meetings while maintaining close treatment team relationships: Saying one thing in each meeting to gently push back but ensuring it is strengths-based for everyone involved (see Clinical Vignette 2).
4. *Advocate for clients with other providers:* You might consult with or attend other clinical or social service appointments with clients if they report feeling belittled by other providers either within or external to your agency.

> **Clinical Vignette 2**
> An Example of Constructively Pushing Back Against Systemic Dehumanization of Clients
>
> During one staffing, a clinician was talking about a female client who engaged in sex work professionally and had started using substances again after a period of abstinence. He shot off a series of one-liners: "She's really off the rails. She lit up her utox like a Christmas tree. She's just out there hookin' again." Everyone laughed, except me. I waited until the laughter died down and noted, "With everything she's been through, I think it's really amazing that she's still finding a way to put food on the table for her kids." Everyone looked at each other – slow nods of agreement came, "Yeah, yeah it is," "She's been through a lot of trauma," and "We'll be trying to get her back into groups." Over time, this kind of talk decreased substantially – even among staunchly abstinence-based clinicians. The clinician referred to above even eventually consulted with a harm reduction clinician herself involved in sex work to become more sensitive to his clients' needs moving forward.

To better support our clients on the individual level, we also work to make our treatment systems less punitive and more aligned with harm reduction by consulting and providing our support on larger community- and policy-level harm reduction efforts. On the community level, we have advocated for community-based harm reduction efforts by speaking at the International Overdose Awareness Day, contributing to public service announcements supporting safer consumption sites, sitting on local opioid taskforces, and advocating for community members to be invited to, and compensated for, sitting on panels, presenting alongside us, and speaking to audiences about

In engaging in systems-level advocacy, we support other local, state, and national harm reduction efforts that benefit our clients

their experiences and their community's needs. On the policy level, we have worked with state legislators to draft a bill removing the long-standing requirement that all state-funded substance use treatment is abstinence-based (Washington State HB1768), and we have supported decriminalization efforts personally and professionally (sitting on state committees, reviewing and providing feedback regarding bills under consideration, signing on to petitions, contacting representatives). Even though, as clinicians, we are most active on the individual level of harm reduction, we can and should be furthering this work on other levels as well.

Avoiding Collusion With More Oppressive Entities

As harm reductionists, we strive to minimize our setting's, or at least our own, collusion with entities that can exact punishment on our clients and community members. This can be a challenging goal, because your clinic or treatment agency might have a contract and thus make financial gains in working with clients mandated by other agencies (e.g., the criminal justice system, child protective services). At the same time, we also recognize that we have some systemic power to advocate on our clients' behalf, and our clients often value this aspect of our power and privilege. But how to advocate within the system without inadvertently contributing to our own clients' oppression can be more challenging that it seems.

> **We leverage our power to support clients, resist oppressive systems, and are transparent about our limitations**

Here are some thoughts that have helped us differentiate from, and make decisions about, how we work with outside entities (see Box 9 for key takeaways). First, we acknowledge that our unique role and responsibilities as psychologists and, more specifically, substance use treatment professionals will have different priorities and obligations from those of other professionals who work with our clients. As psychologists, our primary responsibility is to our clients, whereas other services may be primarily responsible for ensuring other priorities are met, such as public safety (criminal justice) or children's well-being (child protective services) in a given community. That said, our ethical standards also indicate our responsibility for safeguarding the welfare of the larger community, and our state laws often indicate we are mandated reporters. Thus, if we learn about our client's intent to harm themselves or others, we are required to report it through pathways outlined by our own professional ethical codes and state laws. Further, our work as harm reduction clinicians (and psychologists) should be healing for the client – beneficent and nonmaleficent. The general principles outlined by the American Psychological Association also state that our "professional judgments and actions may affect the lives of others, [so we] are alert to and guard against personal, financial, social, organizational, or political factors that might lead to misuse of [our] influence" (American Psychological Association, 2017). Thus, we must ensure our services do not cause more harm than good. We know incarceration and separation of families, often unwittingly abetted by treatment professionals reporting simply on active substance use, have often caused devastating intergenerational harm and historical trauma. Finally, and purely pragmatically, contracted services with substance use treatment providers are often unnecessarily duplicative: It is not uncommon for external entities to require clients to disclose substance use and provide urine samples for toxicology testing in their own facilities.

> **Box 9**
> **Unwitting Collusion With Mass Incarceration and Family Separation**
>
> As a profession, substance use treatment providers have often been unwittingly colluding with mass incarceration and family separation. Here are ways to identify potential collusion, and differentiate and put the client first.
> - Other entities have different roles in the system. If we are co-opted, we should resist by citing our own profession's ethical codes and/or state laws defining our role.
> - As harm reduction clinicians (and psychologists), we are ethically (and sometimes legally) obligated to put the client first, including their welfare, privacy, and confidentiality. This is different from other entities where other goals may be prioritized (e.g., public safety, child welfare).
> - We have our own pathways to mandated reporting and reducing potential community harm. We do not need to take on the pathways of other entities as our own.
> - We do not necessarily need to duplicate and report on services other entities already do (e.g., routine urine toxicology, self-reported use).

How does this translate into practice? In the HaRT track at our institution, we decided against using the typical reporting form for mandated clients. Instead, we discuss with our clients our positionality in the system in relationship to other entities with whom we have contracts. We discuss the potential pros and cons of our provision of information about the client to other entities, listen to clients' perspectives, and formulate a plan together with clients. Thus, with a clearly stated release of information and Health Insurance Portability and Accountability Act (HIPAA) authorization, we can communicate with other entities to indicate what information we decided with the client we could provide. Typically, this has included a letter outlining what HaRT generally entails (i.e., mindset, heartset, and components), that the client had committed to once weekly meetings to engage in HaRT, and their attendance record to indicate treatment exposure (see sample letter in Appendix 2). We have also gone to court or written to judges and probation officers to indicate client involvement in evidence-based HaRT. Finally, it bears repeating that we try to avoid punitive collusion and service or role duplication; thus, we do not provide urine toxicology reports or disclose clients' self-reported substance use, because they are not directly relevant to our primary goals (harm reduction and QoL improvement), and because we do not want to be complicit with punitive systems.

In HaRT, we carefully consider how information to external entities could lead to harm for our clients

Some colleagues have been concerned about taking this stand, wondering if it would cost them contracts or clients. In our experience, some judges, housing providers, social workers with child protective services, and probation or parole officers are relieved to hear HaRT is an evidence-based approach and one that clients are invested in. Because many of our clients have been considered "recidivists" in the system, some entities have even indicated a preference for harm reduction approaches to support clients' treatment engagement and unique recovery trajectories and to avoid a pile-up of repeat offenses they have to serially manage simply on the basis of substance use and relapse. Further, as noted above, our omission of urine toxicology reports and self-reported substance use often does not present

Some external entities are open to non-abstinence-based approaches, especially for clients who are considered system "recidivists"

a problem, because other entities are already monitoring clients' substance use, and/or they focus more on whether clients commit a crime versus engage in substance use per se.

3.3 Assessment of HaRT Efficacy on Key Outcomes

HaRT involves assessment of various process and outcome variables, which can be streamlined for faster-paced settings (e.g., high-volume case management, emergency department clinicians) or expanded (e.g., private psychotherapy, research) as needed and desired.

3.3.1 Assessment of Safer-Use Strategies and Harm Reduction Goal Setting

The SHaRE form can be used to record clients' generation and achievement of harm reduction goal setting and safer-use strategies

The Safer-Drinking and Harm Reduction Efforts (SHaRE) form (Figure 5) is an open-ended grid created for use in HaRT sessions that captures client-endorsed harm reduction goals and safer-use strategies as well as progress made toward them (Collins, Clifasefi, et al., 2019). We have used the SHaRE in various formats: as a paper-and-pencil form inserted in hardcopy client records, in online surveys and databases, and within clinic-based electronic health records (EHRs), depending on the setting and resources.

As discussed in greater detail in Chapter 4, clinicians elicit harm reduction goals (i.e., "What would you like to see happen for yourself during the next week?") and safer-use strategies (i.e., "Which of the strategies we discussed would you be willing to try out over the next week?") using open-ended questions and then record clients' responses on the SHaRE so that a single harm reduction goal and safer-use strategy appears in each cell of the appropriate part of the grid.

For example, a client might indicate an interest in "getting back to work." As shown in Figure 5 and Figure 6 and in Section 4.1.3, the clinician then helps the client develop a goal that is one step they can make toward such larger, existential goals. Weekly goals focus on reducing substance-related harm and/or improving QoL, are precise, and are specified in time and place. In the example used in Figure 5 and Figure 6, the stepwise client goal is to talk to their case manager during their upcoming appointment this Thursday at 3:00 p.m. to learn how to connect with a vocational counselor. We record the smaller goals to be achieved in the next week or until the next session, with the larger goals they serve placed in parentheses *after* the session-to-session goals (see Figure 5).

Similarly, clinicians should work with clients to separate out goals if clients indicate compound goals (e.g., "I need to call my case manager so they can drive me to my court date. I really gotta make that court date") should likely be recorded as (1) call case manager to arrange transportation to court date and (2) attend court date.

SHaRE Form

Participant's Stated Goals (week 1)	Week 2 assessment of week 1 goals	
	Progress y/n	Achieved y/n
1 Talk to case manager about voc counseling – Thurs 3pm (getting back to work)		
2		
3		
4		
5		
6		
7		
Week 2 notes on progress towards goals since week 1:		

Figure 5
Safer-Drinking and Harm Reduction Efforts (SHaRE) form for harm reduction goal setting. This form is available in Appendix 6 for personal/professional use.

In the next session, clinicians will check in with clients to assess whether they achieved (yes/no) or made progress toward (yes/no) their stated harm reduction goals or implemented the safer-use strategy (yes/no) set during the prior sessions (see Figure 6).

SHaRE Form

Participant's Stated Goals (week 1)	Week 2 assessment of week 1 goals	
	Progress y/n	Achieved y/n
1 Talk to case manager about voc counseling – Thurs 3pm (getting back to work)	y	y
2		
3		
4		
5		
6		
7		
Week 2 notes on progress towards goals since week 1:		

Figure 6
Safer-Drinking and Harm Reduction Efforts (SHaRE) form at first follow-up.

We have conducted studies to better understand generation, achievement, and application of harm reduction goals and safer-use strategies (Alawadhi et al., 2023; Collins, Grazioli, et al., 2015; Fentress et al., 2021; Grazioli et al., 2015). This research has indicated that participants often generate an increasing number of goals and safer-use strategies over the course of HaRT. Even initially, participants report high levels of achievement of goals and application of safer-use strategies, and this proportion stays steady or even increases across the treatment course. Greater goal generation of any kind is associated with greater improvements in physical health-related QoL, and the presence of alcohol-specific harm reduction goals is associated with greater reductions in peak drinking amounts, as well as abstinence (Fentress et al., 2021). Safer-use strategies tend to be employed more by participants who are using more heavily and count on those strategies to stay safer and healthier. When participants endorse safer-use strategies that aim to either keep them healthier when drinking or to reduce their drinking, we have sometimes found in our research that their alcohol-related harm decreases in accordance (Alawadhi et al., 2023).

3.3.2 Assessment of Substance Use Outcomes

Be sure to regularly assess substance use and substance-related harm

We recommend *assessment of substance use quantity, frequency,* and *route of administration* at each session, as well as substance-related harm once monthly. In clinical situations, we recommend assessing many of these aspects of use in the context of clients' substance use narrative, which is elicited as a key component of the treatment (see Section 4.1.3 for more detail). Namely, clinicians will start with an open-ended question: "Tell me a little bit about your substance use," or "What did your substance use look like this past week?" As clients share their narrative, clinicians can ask follow-up questions: "What else have you used?" or "What else?" until the client indicates no further substance use. At the end of this elicited narrative, clinicians should be able to document the clients' frequency of use (e.g., number of days of use), quantity of use (e.g., amount used each day), and route of administration (e.g., snorting, smoking, injecting, ingesting, anal injection or "booty bumping," and/or anal application or "hooping"). Ancillary aspects include clients' set (e.g., motivations, affect, and expectancies around use) and setting (e.g., environment, other people involved), which can play an important role in relative risk assessment and in shaping the personalized relative risk hierarchies, described in Section 4.1.3.

With quantity of substances consumed, we recommend you record whatever metrics are most relevant for the specific substance and can be assessed consistently across sessions. For many substances, these metrics will be grams, ounces, or dollar amount spent. For smoking, clinicians will record number of cigarettes or other relevant measures of tobacco or nicotine use (e.g., vape cartridges, number of cigars or cigarillos). For alcohol use, clinicians will record number of standard alcoholic drinks (i.e., 12-oz beer 5% ABV, 5-oz glass of wine 12% ABV, 1.5-oz hard liquor 40% ABV). If you work with a sizable number of clients with AUD, we recommend using the Blood Alcohol Concentration Calculation System (BACCUS), which is a free standard drink calculator created at the University of New Mexico (https://casaa.unm.edu/code/software.html).

In research studies or situations that require more measurement precision, we recommend validated measures, including the following: We have used the Alcohol and Substance-Use Frequency Assessment portion of the Addiction Severity Index (ASI; McLellan et al., 1992). To measure quantity of alcohol use, our research team has developed and used the Alcohol Quantity Use Assessment (AQUA) to more precisely capture alcohol consumption that does not necessarily conform to traditional standard drink measures (e.g., sharing bottles, consuming beverages from large-volume containers [e.g., 16-, 24-, and 40-oz bottles and cans], and use of nontraditional alcohol forms [e.g., high-gravity malt liquor, craft beer, nonbeverage alcohol]). In case clients need a memory hook, we recommend the psychometrically sound *Timeline Followback* (Sobell & Sobell, 1992), which is a set of monthly calendars that allows for retrospective evaluation of substance use for each day of a set period of time. This measure can be used to aggregate various outcomes of interest, including number of days of use, peak use day, average quantity per day of use, etc. Clients could also keep a daily use diary if they have trouble remembering their consumption from week to week.

The Short Inventory of Problems for Alcohol and Drugs (SIP-AD) is a 15-item, Likert-scale questionnaire that measures social, occupational, and psychological substance-related harm experienced over the past 30 days (see Appendix 3). Responses can be summed and placed along its nonnormed scale of 0–45 as a relative measure of harm reduction over the course of treatment (Miller et al., 1995). We highly recommend using this measure across all clients as the primary and universal assessment of substance-related harm, because we have seen the most consistent treatment improvement on it across our studies. The SIP score is also the primary outcome that will be presented in the assessment and tracking component outlined in Section 4.1.3. Additionally, we find it helpful to elicit from clients, and then collaboratively track, other measures of substance-related harm that they feel are relevant to their specific recovery trajectory (e.g., number of seizures, falls, blackouts, or overdoses in the past 30 days or since the last session).

3.3.3 Lab Testing and Biomarkers

In medical settings, it can be helpful to collect and test serum and urine samples to assess the impact of substances on the body through biomarkers. A serum metabolic panel that includes liver transaminases and liver function tests (e.g., AST, ALT, albumin, bilirubin total and direct, and gamma-glutamyl transferase [GGT]) can provide snapshots of liver and renal functioning. Urine tests might include complete urinalysis (UA) to further assess renal functioning.

Outside of research trials, we typically do not recommend the systematic use of breathalyzers or urine toxicology tests because these send clients a message that abstinence continues to be prioritized, which is incongruent with the harm reduction mindset and heartset undergirding HaRT. More important, urine toxicology testing can be stressful for clients who have

Biomarkers of substance use and substance-related harm can make feedback and tracking more impactful and multidimensional

We do not recommend compulsory use of breathalyzers and urine toxicology testing

experienced urine toxicology testing in prior treatment and criminal justice settings that often use punitive and humiliating means of collecting samples and of using. There are, of course, some clinically necessary exceptions to this rule, such as testing for opioids before prescribing naltrexone, to avoid triggering opioid withdrawal.

However, when we are conducting larger program evaluations or research studies, we have found it helpful to assess quantitated level of ethyl glucuronide (EtG; Wurst et al., 2003) or conduct unmonitored urine toxicology for other substances to bioverify self-reported use and/or show that some proportion of research participants are reducing use, which is often a goal for participants. In these contexts, we are very careful to outline to research participants exactly what will be measured in the urine toxicology tests and be very clear that we will not be sharing that information under any circumstances with any outside entities. This is an important step, given the understandable anxiety many people who use substances have around urine toxicology testing.

In harm reduction treatment for smoking, we have used handheld equipment to measure carbon monoxide parts per million in exhaled air (CO; Micro+basic Smokerlyzer; Bedfont Scientific Ltd., Kent, England) and spirometry (i.e., forced expiratory volume; LungLife; Bedfont Scientific Ltd., Kent, England). Of these, we find CO measurement the most helpful, as it is easily obtained and versatile as an outcome measure. It may be used as biochemical verification of self-reported smoking as well as a clear and highly responsive indicator of reduced smoking-related harm (i.e., CO is eliminated from the body within 8-12 hrs after the last cigarette smoked). These measurements can be easily integrated into harm reduction feedback and tracking for clients to monitor their reductions in smoking-related harm. This measure has clinical impact for clients because most clients are aware and have some experience of CO (e.g., toxic element of car exhaust) and its potential harms. As clients reduce their use of combustible tobacco products, seeing CO level decrease so quickly can be an incredibly reinforcing aspect of harm reduction treatment for smoking.

3.3.4 Measures of QoL Outcomes

General health-related QoL measures may not be sensitive enough in the context of HaRT

We have used various QoL measures in our research projects, with varying levels of success. To date, the only measure that has registered statistically significant change through the evidence-based harm reduction treatment approaches we discuss in this book has been the physical health-related QoL scale of the Short Form-12 (SF-12; Ware et al., 1996). The SF-12 is a well-validated, 12-item questionnaire that assesses various aspects of physical and mental health-related QoL. It is, however, less accessible given it is a proprietary measure that must be purchased for access to scoring templates.

3.3.5 Measures for Utilization and Cost Analysis

In larger scale program evaluations or research evaluations, we have assessed administrative data on high-cost and publicly funded service utilization (e.g., jail, court system, emergency medical services and/or emergency department use; see Clifasefi et al., 2013, 2017; Collins, Goldstein, Suprasert, et al., 2021; Collins et al., 2017; Collins, Lonczak, et al., 2019; Larimer et al., 2009; Mackelprang et al., 2014). These data can detect reduction of costs to community providers and have been successful in our team's efforts to better understand larger systems utilization and – in the context of positive treatment outcomes in these areas – boost public, policy, and government support for harm reduction programming at the community and policy levels.

Larger evaluations can benefit from the inclusion of measures that reflect system-wide impacts of substance use

3.3.6 Treatment Integrity Materials and Measures

We often supervise students, trainees, and employees, assessing their HaRT adherence and competence, to ensure treatment integrity for our research studies, clinical supervision, and HaRT certification programs. To this end, we have clinicians audio record their sessions so we may review and provide feedback in group supervision. For a more detailed assessment of manual adherence and competence in our research trials, we use *adherence and competence scales* (see Appendices in Collins et al., 2021). The coding system, which was originally based on the COMBINE Study Medical Management Adherence Checklist and coding schema (Miller et al., 2005; Pettinati et al., 2004), consists of seven dimensions to assess delivery of the HaRT content (count of manualized components delivered converted to a proportion) and style (i.e., informativeness, direction, authoritativeness, warmth, manual adherence, avoidance of nonmanualized components). Style dimensions are rated on 7-point Likert scales, ranging from 0 (*absence of the characteristic*) to 6 (*very high levels of the characteristic, within top 10% of clinicians*). However, in purely clinical contexts, we simply review recordings in group supervision/staffing meetings and provide play-by-play feedback to boost adherence.

In research trials, we formally assess treatment integrity, including manual adherence and competence

4

HaRT Implementation

In this chapter, we translate the HaRT mindset and heartset into the day-to-day language of clinical practice and provide a complete HaRT protocol to use as a step-by-step guide through the three primary components (i.e., collaborative tracking of client-preferred metrics, elicitation of harm reduction and QoL goals, and discussion of safer-use strategies). Finally, we provide some auxiliary components for use in more medicalized settings.

4.1 Method of Approach

4.1.1 HaRT Mindset

Transparency About Your Role

> The HaRT mindset is transparent, pragmatic and focuses on a mutual understanding of clients' relative risks and safety

> Provide a treatment rationale and informed consent process to define HaRT and your role as a harm reductionist

First and foremost, you need to start with transparency about who you are, what HaRT is, what system you are functioning in, your positionality in the system, and how you will be applying HaRT within the setting, including what you can and cannot do to advocate for the client.

Starting with informed consent both at the beginning of treatment and on an ongoing basis, you want to clearly state your treatment rationale for HaRT. Here is an example script you can use and tailor to your professional identity and the system you are working in. You should prepare a clear rationale in advance, and you may integrate your HaRT operationalization into your practice or clinic paperwork, as needed.

"I am a [title, job description] at [xx]. I do harm reduction treatment. This is a different approach to substance use treatment. When we meet, I will not require, ask, or advise you to stop or cut down your substance use or change your use in any way you do not want to. Instead, my focus is to understand what your goals, intentions, or visions for your future are, and I will work with you to help you move towards those. I will also help you assess the relative risks of your substance use behavior so you can make scientifically informed decisions about your substance use. Ultimately, in harm reduction, we want to help people and communities reduce their substance-related harm – the problems people experience due to substance use – and improve their quality of life on their own terms and on their own timeline. How does that sound to you? (or, What questions do you have?)"

Co-Learning About Relative Risks

As we have noted, HaRT requires that harm reduction clinicians are well-informed about substance use and its relative risks. You must understand the relative risks of the various substances your clients are using, as well as the relative risks of their route of administration (see examples in Figures 7, 8, and 9 and more resources in Further Reading section).

With a foundation in harm reduction and what safer use can look like, you will enter into conversation with your clients. As you transition to the HaRT practice, you might notice that your clients share more openly about what they are using and how. You will want to engage in this co-learning process with your clients (see Box 10). You do not need to angle yourself as the expert but listen with curiosity and be ready with affirmations for their engagement in safer-use strategies as they naturally come up.

Harm reduction clinicians co-learn about relative risks with clients and share collective knowledge to inform safer use

> **Box 10**
> **How to Effectively Engage in Co-Learning About Relative Risk**
>
> - Get to know relevant relative risk hierarchies.
> - Learn from clients and then check that info with authoritative sources.
> - Do not provide a relative risk monologue.
> - Instead, drop in bits of psychoeducation on relative risks throughout the session, paired with affirmations and strengths-based reflections.
> - Do ask for permission to provide info on relative risks if a person mentions engaging in or wanting to engage in a riskier behavior.

During these more casual discussions, we recommend avoiding monologues on relative risks. Instead, we make discussion of relative risks more conversational, dropping small bits of psychoeducation throughout the session when and where it is relevant. For example, if your client indicated they have moved from injecting to smoking heroin, you can offer an affirmation and then drop in the psychoeducation to clarify why you are affirming their behavior (see Box 11). This is especially effective paired with strengths-based reflections and open-ended questions to elicit and reinforce stories about safer use.

> **Box 11**
> **Example of Dropping in Psychoeducational Information**
>
> "It so great that you achieved your goal of switching from injecting to smoking heroin this past week! You know, smoking heroin is much safer than injecting because it bypasses the risks of injection, like passing on HIV or Hep C or getting an abscess. So, way to keep yourself safer and healthier this week! Tell me more about how that went."

Of course, then you will want to check with authoritative sources regarding any safer-use strategies that clients are bringing to your sessions that might be unfamiliar to you. This is an important step that cannot be overlooked. Clients often intend to engage in safer use, but due to the lack of mainstream and accessible information sources, they might not have the most accurate or up-to-date information. Even traditionally authoritative sources can get it wrong and do harm. For example, many smokers we have worked with have relayed that they continued smoking due to their physician's [harmfully erroneous] assertion that electronic cigarettes and vaping are more dangerous than smoking. (Please review Section 1.3.3 if you need more information about some research debunking this falsehood.)

If you do learn that your client is engaging in riskier use, we recommend you ask their permission to share some information. For example, your client brings up that they are not able to reliably access new safer-use equipment, but they note making an effort to clean their existing equipment, namely with lemon juice. You might say, "I know you're doing everything you can to use more safely, which is awesome. I have some additional information for you and am hoping I can share it? [Client affirms.] Cleaning your equipment with lemon juice can actually be riskier, because it can introduce bacterial or fungal infections. If you have access to bleach, that would be a safer option if you can't get clean equipment. What do you think?" You can then elicit any questions or troubleshoot barriers to safer use.

Internalizing Relative Risk Hierarchies

As you learn your foundational information about relative risks and safer use, you can start to build relative risk hierarchies that are most relevant to the client base you are seeing. Then, you can go on to affirm a safer behavior and drop in the psychoeducation about what makes that specific behavior safer. Conversely, you can more readily identify if a person is moving into less safe territory and provide corrective information – again, with permission.

Over the years of working with people experiencing homelessness and severe AUD with physiological dependence, we have set up a relative risk hierarchy (see Figure 7) with an eye toward what can precipitate worsening alcohol withdrawal symptoms (e.g., after reducing to lower ABV beer, a client returns to higher ABV malt liquor) or blackouts (e.g., consuming hand sanitizer "cocktails" where mixers mask the flavor and thus perceived concentration of this high-ABV product).

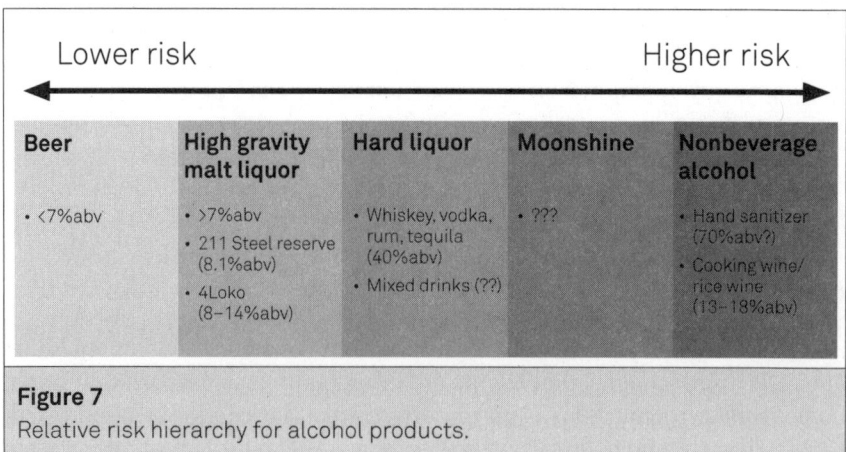

Figure 7
Relative risk hierarchy for alcohol products.

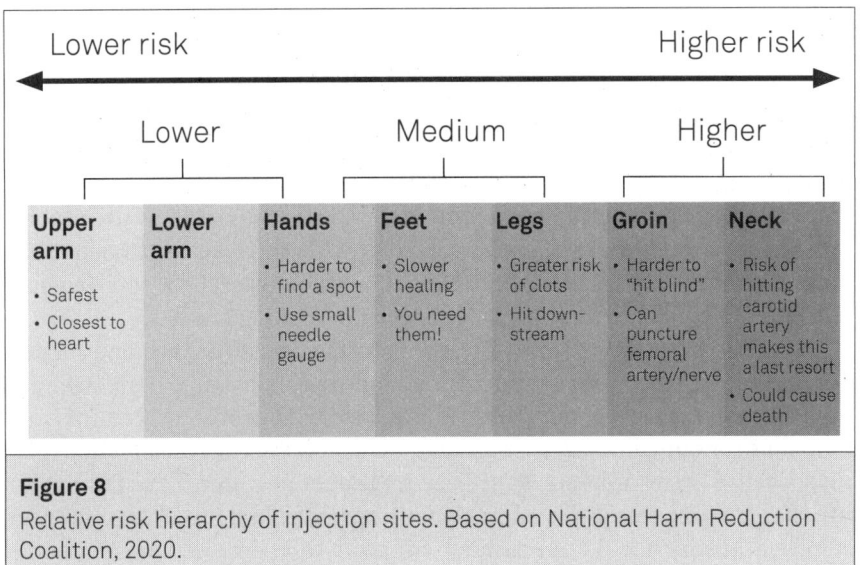

Figure 8
Relative risk hierarchy of injection sites. Based on National Harm Reduction Coalition, 2020.

We were inspired to create the next relative risk hierarchy (see Figure 8) when we read the excellent guide from the National Harm Reduction Coalition called "Getting Off Right" that covers relative risks at each turn of the complex set of medical procedures that is injection drug use (National Harm Reduction Coalition, 2020).

As shown in Figure 9, the relative risk hierarchy for nicotine is relatively simple. As typically used by adults, nicotine itself is a highly addictive and complex, yet relatively harmless stimulant; thus, a focus on less risky means of obtaining nicotine is the most reliable way to reduce risk. Some researchers have estimated that anything that is *not* smoking is about 85% safer than smoking, but even reducing smoking can reduce cardiovascular risks. A complete switchover to chew tobacco is approximately 85% safer, vaping is 95% safer, and nicotine replacement therapy (i.e., patches, gum, lozenges) is 99% safer than smoking (Nutt et al., 2014).

> Create relative risk hierarchies to be prepared for ongoing discussions of relative risks

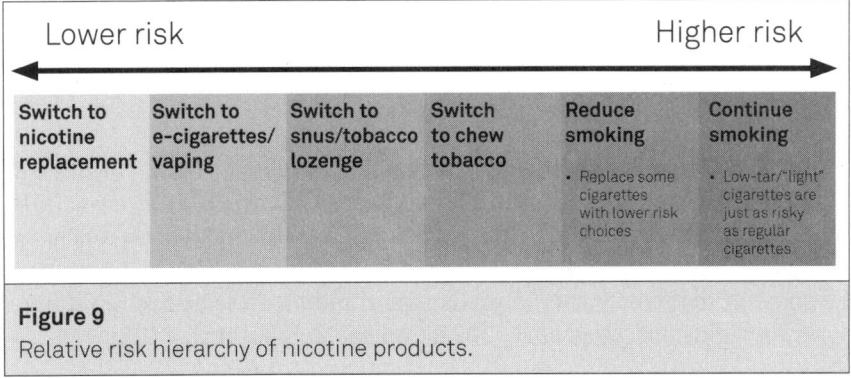

Figure 9
Relative risk hierarchy of nicotine products.

Deferral to Clients' Decision Making

Up to this point, we have talked about your active involvement as a clinician: Providing the HaRT rationale through a transparent informed consent process and engaging in co-learning about relative risks. In this process, the client is inviting you to walk with them on their recovery pathway. You are walking and talking through their experiences with them. They get to a fork in the road where they can make different decisions about their use moving forward. You can ask their permission to provide information to help them make a scientifically informed decision about their use. Then, you step back and defer to your client and their own decision-making process.

> After helping clients assess the relative risks we defer to them to make decisions about their use

It is important at this point to remember that we can engage and support our clients, we can provide information, and we can leverage our power and privilege to advocate for our clients in the system. However, we cannot make decisions for our clients or control their behavior. We raise this point explicitly, because many of us substance use treatment providers have felt implicitly charged with this duty and personally responsible if our clients have not achieved abstinence. Well-intended attempts to coerce or control clients' behavior are usually counterproductive for the client and, in our experience, contribute to clinician burnout (see our rationale in Box 12).

Box 12
Why We Don't Try to Sell the Client on Abstinence or Our Own Agenda

Oftentimes, our training, systems pressures, and our own righting reflex makes us feel a sense of urgency to "sell" the client on a goal we have in mind that we think is in their best interest – typically abstinence or use reduction. We overlook the fact that they might not be ready, willing, or able to "buy" what we are selling. In fact, in substance use treatment, we *usually* start with our agenda without asking the client what they want to see happen for themselves. Thus, we introduce discord into the therapeutic relationship as a matter of course, even feeling justified in doing so. We do this despite the fact both clinical experience and research studies show that it is statistically rare for people who use substances to even want to go to treatment, much less to be told what to do and unquestioningly submit to our suggestions. Some might take this as a challenge they will meet head-on, and the situation can escalate. Others will withdraw from treatment either literally (e.g., "I never graduated [treatment]. I think I've been to like 18 of them. And I never graduated, not one of them") or emotionally (e.g., "People that are forced into treatment don't tend to listen on what's being preached to them" (excerpted from Nelson et al., 2022). Regardless, we have lost the client through our sales pitch for abstinence. And we slowly burn ourselves out or burn our clients out with our failure in Sisyphean salesmanship.

In contrast, our research on harm reduction has shown that client-directed HaRT is associated with reduced use and harm (Collins, Clifasefi, et al., 2019; Collins, Duncan, et al., 2021). Moreover, both intrinsic motivation for change and client leadership in determining recovery pathways have been shown to be some of the most powerful predictors of reduced use and reduced harm (Collins, Goldstein, King, et al., 2021; Collins, Malone, et al., 2012).

4.1.2 HaRT Heartset

In this section, we will discuss the HaRT heartset, or our *way of being with* ourselves and our clients, as well as ways to embody the heartset through words and actions.

Values

The HaRT heartset both aligns with values common to client-centered care and expands them to become more transformative and advocacy-oriented. We review the heartset values briefly before we show how they are integrated into clinical practice. First, there is sense of *acceptance* and support of the client, or from a humanistic or motivational interviewing standpoint, unconditional positive regard (Miller & Rollnick, 2013; Rogers, 1957). Harm reduction clinicians have a sense of *compassion* – or "feeling with" the client, which, depending on the clinician's spiritual or clinical practice, is well-paired with lovingkindness (*Mettā* or *Matrī* in the Buddhist and Vedic traditions), or a desire to remove clients' suffering (Bibeau et al., 2016). This sense inspires *flexibility* and *responsiveness* to the client and their state, including their level of intoxication in session, cognitive functioning, and disabilities (see Clinical Vignette 3 for a clinical example).

> **Clinical Vignette 3**
> Flexibility in HaRT
>
> Due to his medical history including multiple traumatic brain injuries, regular seizures, and alcohol-related cognitive impairment, one of our clients could not remember his alcohol consumption from week to week to complete our regular substance use assessments. At his suggestion, we provided him with a number for texting his daily use. By accommodating his disability on his own terms, we were making his treatment more accessible and engaging.

HaRT values are grounded in *cultural humility* – a lifelong-learner approach entailing openness to, curiosity about, and commitment to uplifting clients' values, ways, and priorities in the face of clients' systems-level oppression (Tervalon & Murray-Garcia, 1998). We also appreciate the cultural *competemility* model (Campinha-Bacote, 2019), in which there is a balance between cultural competence and cultural humility. Within this framework, we learn as much as we can about the communities we work with – population-level demographics; health inequities; cultural beliefs, values, and practices; preferred and effective treatments – *and* we do not assume this general cultural knowledge will hold true for every individual we encounter. Instead, we carefully pay attention to what is said and unsaid, learning from our clients on their own terms and as they craft strengths-based narratives for their own benefit instead of our own. We recognize our own identities and values and consciously set them aside so we may be open to clients' ways, values, knowledge, and strengths, and we commit to elevating them in our work. We recognize our power and privilege and the inequities our clients face, and we push back in our systems of care on their behalf.

On this note, the HaRT heartset requires we engage in systems-level *advocacy* for our clients and help clients engage in self-advocacy as well.

The HaRT heartset entails cultural humility, acceptance, compassion, flexibility, advocacy

Systems-level advocacy means speaking up on behalf of clients within our systems of care, attending other appointments with them where they have felt marginalized (see Clinical Vignette 4), or shaping policy locally or on the larger public health level. In supporting clients' ability to self-advocate, we connect clients with local harm reduction organizations – preferably those that are community-based and user-led (e.g., National Urban Survivor's Union, People's Harm Reduction Alliance, Never Use Alone, VOCAL). These can foster clients' sense of community and provide opportunities for clients to volunteer, support their community, and engage in policy advocacy.

> **Clinical Vignette 4**
> Advocating for Clients in Our Systems of Care
>
> One client had high treatment adherence: He regularly took his prescribed suboxone and hypnotics for sleep and attended both group and individual treatment sessions. He continued to smoke the same amount of heroin every day and did not use other substances. When he admitted to his addiction psychiatrist that he was still smoking heroin, the psychiatrist told the client he would no longer prescribe the hypnotic for sleep if the client did not stop smoking heroin. After receiving this information, the client felt he could not be honest about his substance use with his addiction psychiatrist. He began experiencing increased anxiety symptoms, including intrusive thoughts and insomnia. He worried about the threat of losing his sleep medication, its potential effects on his sleep and his ability to manage his daily treatment routine. Consultation with other harm reduction physicians indicated there was little safety concern given the client's history and stable, ongoing use. The clinician offered to attend his appointment with him and advocate should the addiction psychiatrist deny his prescription. The addiction psychiatrist was pleased the client was so engaged as to involve his team. No questions were asked; he wrote the prescription and did not make the threat again. A year later, the client, with his sleep intact, stopped using heroin, but on his own terms and timeline.

Finally, HaRT emphasizes a *holistic* and *transformative* approach to substance use treatment. Specifically, harm reduction clinicians care about clients' growth and thriving as a whole person, including and beyond their substance use behavior. In place of striving for abstinence, we support clients in achieving whatever can help them reduce their substance-related harm and improve their QoL. Positive changes in QoL can be as simple as going to the library more often or as complex as reconnecting with estranged family members. You will see this striving for holistic and transformative change become a positive routine that reshapes your understanding of your client and their own self-image as you provide week-by-week support of client-driven harm reduction goals. This ongoing process supplants the long-standing tradition of provider-driven, abstinence-based or use reduction goals in substance use treatment.

How to Build a Strong Foundation for the Heartset

To do this work day after day requires compassion – for yourself as a clinician and also for your clients. When we first started conducting trainings in harm reduction, however, we realized we could not explain to clinicians how to tap into compassion. We started to question whether we really knew how to tap into compassion ourselves. Despite the fact it was already a buzzword in the 2010s, this was not something that had been cultivated in us through our psychology programs in the 1990s.

And so, we googled it, of course. We found talks on compassion with speakers exhorting us to imagine our way into someone else's experience. In one such talk, the speaker pleaded with the audience, "Imagine! You are a 9-year-old. In Myanmar. And your family has just lost everything in a devastating earthquake!" Honestly, we found we could not imagine that at all. Even as we tried, it was challenging to cognitively position ourselves to feel someone else's pain when the starting point was so far from our own lived experiences.

We learned we were not alone. Scientific studies have shown that it is not easy to "imagine" or think one's way into compassion for and kindness to others (Weng et al., 2013). Even when you can, doing so is more connected to empathy, or taking on others' emotional states and perspectives, which can even lead to increased negative affect (Klimecki et al., 2013). Since the 2010s, the scientific literature has shown that building compassion, which is sensing others' emotional states paired with a desire to reduce suffering, effectively builds not only affective empathy but also *accurate* empathy, altruism, self-care, and affect regulation (Bibeau et al., 2016).

One study in particular gave us some insight into the how and why behind compassion. Weng and colleagues (2013) showed they could train participants in lovingkindness or *mettā* meditation to build their compassion like a muscle. In this study, participants were randomized into two groups. One group engaged in 2 weeks of daily, 30-minute lovingkindness meditations in which they sent golden light from their heart and good wishes (e.g., happiness, joy, ease, and freedom from suffering) to a loved one, themselves, neutral parties, and people with whom they had experienced conflict. The second group engaged in cognitive reappraisal exercises, including imagining themselves in someone else's shoes. Participants were then asked to play a videogame in which they needed to redistribute wealth to victims of fairness violations. The participants who were engaged in compassion or lovingkindness meditation more equitably distributed the wealth to the victims than participants engaged in cognitive reappraisal.

Our encouragement for harm reduction clinicians to practice meditation and lovingkindness meditation has increased with our understanding of the importance of embodied and socially engaged means of building compassion in increasing empathy, decreasing emotional reactivity, and preventing burnout. For these reasons, we highly recommend cultivating whatever compassion-building practices best fit your background, values, and lifestyle.

Communicating With HaRT

Communicating with a HaRT heartset entails starting the conversation centering the client; using a strengths-based, harm reduction style in administering the three HaRT components (to be covered in Section 4.1.3) in your sessions; and managing discord, intoxication, and escalation with compassion.

> Compassion for ourselves and our clients through lovingkindness practices is key to the HaRT heartset

> How we communicate with clients conveys the HaRT heartset

Starting the Conversation

In our trainings, we typically introduce attendees to communication that upholds the HaRT heartset using two basic role plays (see Table 2). In both role plays, one person plays the clinician, and the other plays the client. The clinician introduces three prompts and waits for the client to respond, not adding to or taking away from the written content:

Table 2
Abstinence-Based Versus Harm Reduction Role Plays in HaRT Trainings

Role Play 1: Abstinence-based approach	Role Play 2: HaRT approach
• Given your current health problems, I would strongly advise you to stop [drinking/using xx substance].	• Please tell me a little bit about your alcohol and drug use.
• Have you ever stopped [drinking/using xx substance] before?	• What are some things you like about using [alcohol/other drugs]?
• Have you ever gone to AA/12-step program?	• What kinds of concerns do you have about your [alcohol/other drug] use?

Once our attendees have gone through both role plays, we review as a group what it was like to participate in them. What were the differences in how the clinician and client "felt" in both of them? What role play did attendees gravitate toward?

Every training elicits different responses to the prompts. However, relatively universally, attendees have indicated that the prompts in Role Play 1 felt more abrupt, uncomfortable, and judgmental – for both the client and clinician roles. Some attendees have immediately noted that the prompts in Role Play 1 were all closed-ended questions, which even linguistically limits the client to dichotomous, yes/no responses and makes it harder to know what the client is really thinking.

However, many attendees have reported more of an affective response to Role Play 1. At one recent training, the attendee playing the client reported feeling despondent and hopeless about their clinician's ability to understand where they were coming from: "I said, 'Okay. Um, thank you. I'll do that.' But the authentic feeling that I was having was, 'Well, my story is more complicated than what you're saying, and I feel like if I say anything, you're just going to tell me that I have to stop, and we're not really going to have much of a conversation about it. So, I'm just going to smile and say, 'Thank you!' so I can get out of this.'"

Another training attendee responded, "If I was the client, especially if it was – even if it wasn't the first time meeting this person – I would just never want to come back, and I would just go somewhere else."

Training attendees are often surprised to learn that both Role Plays 1 and 2 were real-life counseling situations we observed through our field research. In fact, Role Play 1, shown in Clinical Vignette 5, did not play out in a way any counselor would have intended:

> **Clinical Vignette 5**
> Real-Life Example of the Clinical Aftermath of Assuming an Abstinence-Based Perspective for a Client
>
> Counselor: Have you ever done AA?
> Client: Oh, yeah.
> Counselor: Right on. What do you think about AA?
> Client: To be honest, I see them as a bunch of Nazis.
> [Silence]

Engaging in Active Listening Throughout HaRT Sessions

To bolster engagement in HaRT, you must engage in reflective, active listening consistently throughout all client communications (see Box 13 for nonverbal communication tips). A helpful set of active listening strategies that we engage in HaRT was established in motivational interviewing (Miller & Rollnick, 2013): the use of open-ended questions, affirmations, reflections, and summary statements (OARS).

Open-ended questions, affirmations, reflections, summary statements are shaped to be strengths-based and harm reduction oriented

> **Box 13**
> **More Than Words: Considering Nonverbal Communication in HaRT**
>
> - Inform yourself about the population you will be working with, consult as necessary, and always proceed with cultural humility.
> - Provide your undivided attention. If you hold the emergency phone or are on-call in your workplace, be sure to let the client know in advance, pause the session if you need to take a call, apologize, and turn your attention fully back to the client.
> - Make your eyes readily available for contact, but not necessarily locking. Depending on the culture a person is from, heavy eye contact and firm handshakes might feel threatening or aggressive.
> - Regardless of whether you are seated or standing, you should be angled across from your client to avoid a perception of "squaring off."
> - Uncross your legs and arms to create an open stance.

There is, however, a key differentiation between the use of OARS in motivational interviewing and in HaRT. Although there are other ways to engage OARS (e.g., counseling with neutrality and equipoise), in motivational interviewing, they are most often highlighted in the context of directional focusing and evocation phases of motivational interviewing (Miller & Rollnick, 2013). Very commonly, they are used to develop discrepancy and resolve it in the direction of positive behavior change, which culminates in what the clinician believes are appropriate goals.

In HaRT, by contrast, OARS are not used to develop discrepancy. Instead, they are used to affirm clients' naturally occurring harm reduction behaviors and encourage the client to consider how they can build on their existing resilience, safer-use strategies, and QoL. They are nearly exclusively focused on affirmative, autonomy-supportive, and strengths-based communication. Below, we provide examples of how to re-vision OARS in HaRT.

Open-ended questions are the Hows, the Whats and the Tell-me-abouts. They are used to elicit stories about clients' current use, pros and cons of use, harm reduction goals, and ideas for safer use. Examples include:
- "Tell me a little about your substance use" and "Tell me the best ways you know to measure and track the harm you experience when you're using" (assessment of substance use and relative risks)
- "What would you like to see happen for yourself?" (elicitation of harm reduction goals)
- "How can you keep yourself safer and healthier when you are using?" (considering safer-use strategies)

Affirmations are ways to affirm the client and their inherent humanity. They should be the first thing our clients encounter; they are meant to express our love and acceptance and welcome our clients in our treatment spaces. For particularly marginalized individuals, affirmations can constitute a corrective emotional experience, contrasting with how they might feel excluded from or overlooked in other spaces. Affirmations do not have to be extensive or written out. They can be as simple as a smile or a "Hello!" Affirmations also help reinforce clients' self-efficacy and autonomy for safer use, because they amplify clients' existing ability to engage in harm reduction and QoL improvement. Affirmations may be as simple as a smile or may be woven together with other OARS into a complex tapestry of affirmation:
- "Good morning!" (simple affirmation)
- "Thanks for coming back today!" (affirmation, reflecting behavior)
- "You smoked heroin instead of injecting it. (Reflection) By doing that, you are eliminating your risk for blood-borne illness transmission and abscesses. (harm reduction psychoeducation) Good for you! (affirmation)"

Reflecting what clients have said is a means of showing you are listening by mirroring back to them their words and/or interpreted meaning. Simple reflections hew closely to clients' own words. These can be helpful early on in a relationship, or if discord arises. For example:
- Client: I wish people would get off my case. I don't think my drinking is that big of a deal.
- Clinician: Your drinking's not a big deal. (staying close to client content)

As the relationship deepens, you may use more complex reflections. You may continue clients' thoughts; hypothesize about affective content, perceived pressures, or underlying motivations; or clarify internally conflicting ideas.
- Client: I wish people would get off my case. I don't think my drinking is that big of a deal.
- Clinician: You're bothered others feel they can make decisions for you. (hypothesizing about perceived pressures)

Simple and complex reflections are fine in HaRT, and we do use them. However, *most* reflections in HaRT should be strengths-based and underscore the client's autonomy, self-efficacy, and resilience. For example:

- Client: I wish people would get off my case. I don't think my drinking is that big of a deal.
- Clinician: You know yourself and your drinking best. (emphasizing the positive – self-knowledge over external pressure)

Using strengths-based, harm reduction reflections, you will find yourself more open to locating sources of resilience in clients, even in statements that would be antithetical to and garner disapproval in abstinence-based modalities. For example:

- Client: Meth helps me focus and take care of business.
- Clinician: You like to be efficient and get things done. (emphasizing the positive – pointing out client's values)

Summaries of clients' responses elicited via strengths-based and harm reduction-oriented OARS may be gathered over the course of the session to help clients review their prior statements in a more compact and organized way. Again, emphasizing what clients are already doing to move toward harm reduction – and underscoring that with affirmations – is key to keeping a positive, strengths-based communication loop going. Over time, this looping repeats and positively reinforces safer-use strategies and client-driven goal setting as well as their connection to clients' experience of harm reduction and QoL improvement.

- "From everything you just told me, I can see you've already incorporated safer-use strategies, like spacing your drinks and eating a meal before you drink. Those steps can help you stay healthier when you drink because both slow alcohol's absorption into your bloodstream. Way to make healthier choices for yourself! How does that feel?"

Conversational Conventions: HaRT Versus Abstinence-Based Treatment

Using OARS with a strengths-based, harm reduction focus can facilitate a break with many conversational conventions encountered in abstinence-based treatment. In Table 3, we expand upon this practice by addressing common situations encountered in substance use treatment settings. We differentiate between a commonly encountered abstinence-based treatment response (the "Don't" column) and a response that is congruent with the HaRT heartset (the "Do" column). While we are not making a moral judgment with the "Don't" column, it includes responses that are not congruent with a HaRT approach. Thus, ensuring the "Dos" listed below take the place of the "Don'ts" facilitates a break with common abstinence-based treatment patterns and tropes to help clients more fully and consistently engage with a HaRT heartset.

> Using strengths-based, harm reduction reflections, you will find yourself more open to locating sources of resilience

Table 3
Key Dos and Don'ts of Harm Reduction Treatment (HaRT)

Don't	Do
Ask back-to-back, closed-ended questions about clients' use and recovery involvement.	*Elicit a story about clients' substance use.*
Why not? This can shut a client down and damage the therapeutic alliance. While you might obtain the answers, you might find you do not get to know your client very well. This can also lead a clinician into the assessment or question-and-answer trap as described by Miller and Rollnick (2013).	Why? Linguistically, this will draw a client out and help you get to know them better. This shows a client you are truly placing their priorities first by starting with their story versus your clinical agenda. Consider open-ended questions to elicit clients' story and fill out your assessments using their narrative. Follow-up prompts can flesh out additional needed details. This will also provide you with more information to complete more of a use landscape, encompassing drug, set, and setting in which clients are using. You will also find you will better understand the clients' relative risks and where potential safer-use strategies and quality-of-life enhancers may be worked in.
Therapist: Did you use cocaine in the past 30 days? Client: Yes. Therapist: The past week? Client: No. Therapist: Did you use marijuana in the past 30 days? Client: Yes. Therapist: The past week? Client: Yes. Therapist: Have you gone to treatment before? Client: Yes. Therapist: Have you gone to AA, NA, CA, etc? Client: Yes.	Therapist: Tell me a little bit about your substance use. Client: My mother started drinking when I was 13. It came to a point that I was drinking with her, and these things I carry within me. These things I would like to share, because a lot of people withhold their inner feelings and what they have lived through. Not sharing or talking about these hurts or whatever it is we go through in life and using alcohol and drugs – that hurt my children deeply. It hurt my family. It hurt my community. And these things I need to talk about.[a]

Table 3 continued

Seize on a client's expressed desire for abstinence.	*Gently question clients' expressed desire for abstinence.*
Why not? Miller and Rollnick (2013) have referred to this as premature focusing, where clinicians might overshoot clients' current motivational state. If clients do not follow through with behaviors in line with the premature focus, they can feel they have ruptured the therapeutic bond or failed at attempted treatment or sobriety. This often leads to treatment attrition. Client: I just gotta quit. Things are out of control, and I can't go back to jail. Therapist: Ok, based on your assessment, in-patient treatment is a good option.	Why? This can help a client explore their reasoning for this statement and potential ambivalence. It also gives the clinician an opportunity to reiterate the HaRT rationale: as a harm reduction clinician, clients do not have to want to stop using to get help. Client: I just gotta quit. Things are out of control and I can't go back to jail. Therapist: Hm, it seems you are feeling a lot of pressure to stop using. Tell me more about that.
Label the client.	*Avoid labels.*
Why not? Some clients self-identify as "addicts" or "alcoholics," particularly if they are a part of a 12-step community. However, even when unintentional, this reduces the person to the substance they are using or the behavior they engage in, which research has shown can be stigmatizing and dehumanizing. This can also introduce discord and lead to a rupture in the therapeutic bond if it overshoots the client's self-assessment. Therapist: You are an alcoholic. Client: No, I am not. "Alcoholic" has not been a diagnostic category since the DSM-II.[b]	Why? This underscores that you see your clients as people first, with all their complexity and humanity. Version 1 (client not involved in 12-step community): Client: I'm just an alcoholic. Therapist: I see you as so much more than your alcohol use. You are a mother, a sister, a daughter, a counselor. Version 2 (client involved in 12-step community): Client: I go to meetings – I know I am an alcoholic. Therapist: You're invested in 12-step, and an important part of your recovery is acknowledging who you are in this way. But I just want you to know I see you as so much more than your alcohol use. You are a whole person to me, and I really appreciate you. So, I won't use that label, but I understand if you want to.

Note. [a] Community member response quoted in Collins et al. 2022. [b] Quoting Susan E. Collins's experience.

Managing Discord and De-Escalation

Discord in the therapeutic relationship is jointly generated by the clinician and larger systemic pressures

In substance use treatment, we have often referred to clients' pushback as "resistant" or "in denial" of the harm they experience due to substance use. There has, however, been growing acknowledgment that discord is not generated solely by the client but is jointly created in the therapeutic relationship (Miller & Rollnick, 2013). As harm reduction clinicians, we need to avoid blaming the client for discord (e.g., describing them as "argumentative," "treatment resistant," or "in denial"). In fact, we even go beyond the therapeutic relationship as the generative source of discord: We recognize the role of our systems and our own positionality in them, which can foster distrust, oppression, and barriers to healing.

We also need to recognize the heightened risk for discord and escalation in HaRT, because we are more likely to be working with clients who are actively experiencing intoxication and withdrawal cycles, which can engender greater impulsivity, lower inhibitions, and, depending on the substance (e.g., alcohol, stimulants), may be associated with greater levels of restlessness, anxiety, or agitation. Keeping that in mind, harm reduction clinicians must pay even more attention to early signs of discord (see Box 14; Miller & Rollnick, 2013).

Box 14
Pay Attention to Early Signs of Discord

Defending: "It's not my fault"; "It's not that bad."

Squaring off: "Who are you to tell me what to do?"; "You have no idea what it's like for me"; "You're wrong about that."

Interrupting: The client may talk over you and say things like "You don't understand"; "You're not hearing me"; "I don't agree."

Disengaging: The person seems to be inattentive, distracted, or ignoring you. Perhaps the client changes the subject and goes off on a tangent. Their eyes glaze over or glance at a clock.

Working with clients who are intoxicated is a key and important aspect of HaRT. We are modeling compassion to our clients and colleagues and demonstrating session-by-session that working with intoxicated clients is not enabling but can serve as a corrective emotional experience for clients who have been turned away in their times of greatest need (see Box 15). In meeting people where they are at, especially when they show symptoms of SUD, we are demonstrating compassion and acceptance in a substantive way and providing support when clients' need it the most.

Managing Discord

If discord arises, stop, check your nonverbals, downshift to simple reflections, apologize for misunderstanding

When you sense discord in the therapeutic relationship, pause and ensure you are engaging in active, reflective listening (Box 14). In particular, you should downshift to simple reflections, hewing closely to the client's words. As relevant, whole-heartedly apologize for misunderstandings on your part or your own or your system's contributions to the situation. It is important for harm reduction clinicians to take responsibility for our role

> **Box 15**
> **Community Consultant, Joey Stanton, on Meeting People Where They're At (Collins, Black Bear et al., 2018)**
>
> It is important to reflect on the fact that no other diagnosable conditions require that a person is symptom-free *before* they are able to engage in treatment. This strange tradition in substance use treatment and how it impacts clients is best described by community consultant, Joey Stanton, who recounts the answer he received when he asked his psychiatrist, "'What do you do when somebody shows up at your office, and they smell like alcohol?' They tell me, 'I reschedule them.' And I tell them, 'You're a fucking asshole.' Period. Why? What's the skin off your back, man? Who told you that that's ok? They don't turn sick people away from hospitals. If you're bleeding, at least they'll stitch you up, at least listen to you for a minute. But [with people who are intoxicated] it's, 'Oh, we're gonna have to reschedule.'"

in discord, because, again, we are part of the same oppressive systems our clients are embedded within and reacting to. Further, we must resist the urge to defend ourselves or the system, to confront a client, or to make attempts to control or change their behavior. Instead, if you notice discord arising, stop, pause, breathe, and focus on positive affirmations for your client. Then, redirect yourself back to the client, remembering that the healing that needs to happen right now is with the client. Although well-intended, the righting reflex creates ineffective, unhelpful pressures for ourselves and our clients that can deepen the discord. Proceed with simple reflections or strengths-based reflections and affirmations until the discord has dissipated.

Managing Escalation

Discord can be a precursor to escalation. In other cases, especially in the context of withdrawal or intoxication with stimulants or alcohol, clients can escalate very quickly without a clear build up from discord. Alternately, clients may present at the clinic for your appointment already in an agitated state. Depending on your setting, you may come across clients involved in physical or verbal altercations in the waiting room of your office or other public space. The situation calls for a skillful response; thus, we will take a moment to understand the escalation process and review how you might proceed in a calm and reflective way.

Before we talk about managing escalation, let's review what is happening when we experience our clients' (and our own) escalation. You might experience shallow breathing, tunnel vision, higher-pitched or faster rate of speech, a rush through your body. This is called the *stress response*, and it is an instinctual process that prepares us for fight-or-flight mode when our lives are threatened.

Let's consider the biology in play: The hypothalamus sends signals to the sympathetic nervous system, which in turn sends out impulses to glands and smooth muscles and tells the adrenal medulla to release stress hormones (i.e., adrenaline and noradrenaline) into the bloodstream. These stress hormones increase heart rate and blood pressure to rally the system against a threat.

Both clients and therapists can escalate due to the fight-or-flight response

The hypothalamus simultaneously activates the adrenal-cortical system. The pituitary gland releases the adrenocorticotropic hormone, which reaches the adrenal cortex and causes the release of about 30 different hormones to help the body manage the threat (Layton, 2005). This fight-or-flight system is very handy when protecting our lives from an immediate physical threat that could most likely result in death – like a charging saber-toothed tiger. Unfortunately, there is a system mismatch. Fight or flight is not the most adaptive response in our complicated, postmodern world because most daily stressors we encounter, including client escalation, require a far more subtle and differentiated response (see Clinical Vignette 6).

> **Clinical Vignette 6**
> Susan E. Collins Observing the Stress Response in Action
>
> A few years ago, Susan was asked to be one of many speakers at an overdose prevention event. It was in a local park. All of the speakers were lined up on the makeshift stage waiting to speak. Midway through the presentations, a person, swaying a bit, wandered up the steps. He seemed confused what we were doing there and appeared intoxicated and disgruntled by our presence. It was awkward because there was a family talking about how they lost a loved one to overdose, and at the same time, this more marginalized individual seemed confused and displaced. Unfortunately, a well-intentioned case manager from a harm reduction–oriented agency approached the man, squared off, puffed out his chest, balled his fists at his side, and said through clenched teeth, "You need to get off this stage now, Sir." Worried about the potential for escalation, Susan approached at an angle and said, "You can – he can – come stand next to me." It was too late. The man seemed to reel from the exchange with the case manager and left the stage. Susan still thinks about that now, and how the community member might have internalized that experience as a rejection or a threat. She is frustrated that she didn't intervene earlier or more effectively. She also felt for this case manager because he probably wished he had made a different decision, but his body had already released the fight-or-flight hormones. He was ready to fight. We have all been there and made these same mistakes. This moment is where we need to stop, take a breath and interrupt the cycle.

To effectively de-escalate, remove the perceived threat with a nonpunitive, validating response

Managing escalation requires that we model the behavior we hope to see

How can we manage client escalation? First, we need to manage our own stress levels. Stay calm, take a deep breath, figure out what is being triggered in you, and acknowledge that to yourself. Know that you can set that aside for a moment to attend to the clients' needs. Turn your expressed emotion down to zero (for an example of this approach in a group setting, see Clinical Vignette 7).

Then, we attend to our clients. (There are some exceptions to this. If clients are armed or are making explicitly violent threats, please follow your site's safety protocols.) We recommend using open, nonthreatening body language – uncross your arms and legs, angle your body to them, be sure to position yourself between the client and the door or other escape route. Within reason, mirror your clients' expressed emotions, except anger, which can trigger escalation. Whether it is due to social modeling or a function of mirror neurons, humans are social creatures, and we tune into and mirror each others' responses. So, and this is key, if you wish for your client to de-

> **Clinical Vignette 7**
> Seema L. Clifasefi's Advice for Group Settings
>
> We try to be very inclusive in our harm reduction groups and not turn anyone away, even if they are intoxicated. We find this works most of the time. Our open door and low-barrier policy works well if we establish group guidelines and values at the beginning of groups, as well as noting that if a person doesn't feel they can follow through with the guidelines that day, they can try again next time. Our door is always open. If a person escalates during the group session, insulting or yelling at another group member or actively using in the group, we will speak gently to address it. One example: "As we all agreed to, in this group, we're working hard to build peaceful, nonviolent community, part of that is not yelling over each other. Let's all take a moment just to catch our breath. Does this still work for everyone?" If it doesn't, we typically will ask if we can check in with someone outside the group for a one-on-one. Oftentimes, people appreciate that.

escalate, model that behavior. Speak low and slow, use their name to help them focus. Seek to understand what concern the client has, engage in active listening, normalize their feelings, and reflect their strengths. As needed, apologize for your own role or the role of the system you represent in their concern. Empathize with their response. Provide a menu of options, and then let the client guide next steps. For example, in a waiting room where a client is escalating, you could offer, "Hello, Joe. Thank you so much for coming in to talk and sticking with us even though you have a lot going on today/you are not happy with having to wait so long/etc. At this point, we could go back to my office to talk more privately or we could take a walk outside. What do you think would be best?" (See Clinical Vignette 7 for strategies in group settings.)

Once you are out of the situation, be sure to take care of yourself in ways that feel good to you. For example, talk about the situation with a trusted colleague (protecting confidentiality), do a critical incident debrief to check in with other staff, and do physical exercise involving cardio to discharge the tension that builds up following stressful events. For longer-term stress management, it is helpful to have some kind of daily or regular practices to manage stress, such yoga, meditation, and fitness routines.

Remember to take care of yourself after engaging in de-escalation!

4.1.3 HaRT Components and Their Integration in Initial and Follow-Up Sessions

Within the framework of the HaRT mindset and heartset, clinicians enact the three concrete HaRT components: (a) collaborative tracking of client-preferred outcome metrics, (b) elicitation of clients' harm reduction goals, and (c) discussion of safer-use strategies. We explain the implementation of these components and their integration with the aforementioned HaRT mindset and heartset in this section to provide a step-by-step guide for successful HaRT sessions with your client.

Initial HaRT Session

The phases of the initial session include the following (three primary HaRT components are in boldface type):
- Opening the session (5 minutes)
- Eliciting clients' reasons for seeking HaRT (5 minutes)
- Explaining the HaRT rationale and providing an orientation to the session (5 minutes)
- **Reviewing substance use assessment and client-led tracking (5 minutes)**
- **Establishing harm reduction goals (10 minutes)**
- **Introducing safer substance use strategies (10 minutes)**
- Wrapping up (5 minutes)

Opening the Session

Greet the client. If possible, offer them light refreshments (e.g., coffee, water, or juice), and thank them for taking the time to meet with you and to work on their own recovery pathway. If your client base includes people who are intoxicated with stimulants or are agitated, having a fidget basket, which includes sensory-based interventions or toys (e.g., pop-its, stress balls and fidget spinners), within clients' reach can be helpful. See Box 16 to prepare for the client's arrival.

Box 16
Honoring Mirror Neurons and Social Learning in Healing

When clients arrive, it is important to turn on your *emotional radar*. In our research and clinical work, we have observed that clients are often sensitive to what they perceive in the person across from them. In essence, we have found that these clients – as all of us – tend to give back what they are given. It is therefore important to show respect, warmth, and model (not intrusively impose) well-placed boundaries from the first intervention contact. The so-called *nonspecific treatment effect* is a powerful intervention and sets the tone for a positive interaction.

Eliciting Clients' Reasons for Seeking HaRT

Inquire about the client's reasons for seeking HaRT: "What brought you here today?" Elicit the client's story using the harm reduction strengths-based OARS and active listening skills. This will help you assess how much clients understand about their own use, their motivation for change, their understanding of HaRT, and their current clinical disposition.

Explaining the HaRT Rationale and Orientation to HaRT

Orienting clients and providing the opportunity to ask questions can help clients feel more comfortable

Introduce yourself and HaRT using your adaptation of the following script: "I am a [title, job description] at [place]. I do harm reduction treatment. Harm reduction treatment is a different approach from the substance use treatment you may have previously encountered. When we meet, I will not require, ask, or advise you to stop or cut down your substance use or change your use in any way you do not want to. Instead, my focus is on understanding what your goals, intentions, or visions for your future are, and I will work to support you in moving toward those. I will also help you assess the relative risks of your substance use behavior so you can make scientifically informed decisions about your substance use. Ultimately, in harm reduction, we want to help people and communities reduce their substance-related harm – the problems people experience due to substance use – and improve their quality of life on their own terms and on their own timeline."

Elicit clients' responses to this by asking an open-ended question, such as, "How does that sound to you?" Then, respond to any questions – theoretical or practical – that may come up.

For the sake of transparency and informed consent, review the overarching timeline for your treatment course so clients have clear expectations about upcoming visits (see Box 17 for suggestions). Discuss the agenda for the initial session specifically and further elicit and respond to clients' questions. If possible, offer ways you can be flexible in providing services that work with their timeframes and schedule. As applicable, ask clients' permission to record the session. Let clients know this is for review in case consultation and is primarily for quality control of your work.

> **Box 17**
> **HaRT Session Intervals and Treatment Course Options**
>
> In our research trials, we have offered four to five HaRT sessions, spaced first weekly and then monthly. In our clinical practice, we have offered 12 weekly treatment sessions, with an option to continue, as desired and needed by the client. When embedded in longer-term, safety-net, and wraparound case management services, we have also offered longer treatment courses, which after 1 year, typically segue into shortened "check-ins" or aftercare sessions spaced at monthly intervals.

Substance Use Assessment, Feedback, and Tracking

Substance Use Assessment. You will next administer clients' substance use assessment measures (e.g., substance use quantity and frequency, substance-related harm, QoL, and/or biomarkers) as reviewed in Chapter 3. We recommend a specific line of questioning below (see Box 18). If the assessment was conducted prior to your interview by a separate assessment staff, skip to the next section ("Assessment Feedback").

> **Box 18**
> **Essential Substance Use Assessment Checklist**
>
> - Elicit clients' stories about their substance use using open-ended questions ("Please tell me a little about your substance use"),
> - Ask follow-up, open-ended questions to fill in any details missing about quantity, frequency, route of administration.
> - Repeat process of open-ended narrative elicitation until all substances are named (e.g., "Thank you for telling me about your alcohol use. What other substances do you use?").
> - At the end of your open-ended assessment, you should have a complete picture of the drug (i.e., substance quantity, frequency, mode of use), set, and setting.
> - Then, administer the SIP (see Appendix 3).
> - Use this combined information to shape what relative risk hierarchies will be in play and how to best measure substance-related harm.

Try to elicit clients' stories around their substance use to complete your assessment, using follow-up questions to fill in any gaps

If you are administering the assessment yourself, we recommend starting out by eliciting clients' narratives about their substance use using open-ended questions and prompts. This will start building a foundation of cultural humility and respect for client autonomy into your therapeutic relationship. You might say, for example, "A lot of us use substances to celebrate the good times or feel better in the bad times. How about you?" or "Tell me a little bit about your substance use" or "What is your substance use like?" If you must complete formal assessments in your practice, try to use their narrative to complete your clinic's or agency's forms. This will help you avoid the checklist-driven assessment process that can introduce discord. You may and should ask follow-up questions to ensure assessment accuracy and completeness. Here are some examples:

- "Thank you for sharing your perspectives on your substance use. I understand you use heroin daily. How much do you typically use each day in dollar amount or grams?" and "How are you using heroin?" (As they answer, be sure you understand if they are snorting, smoking, injecting/slamming, rubbing anally/hooping, anal dosing/booty bumping, because these all of these will change the relative risks/risk hierarchies you will employ.)
- "So far, you have been kind enough to share about your alcohol, cocaine, and cannabis use. What other substances do you use?" Keep asking, "What else?" after they tell you a story about each substance so you do not miss anything inadvertently (see Clinical Vignette 8).

> **Clinical Vignette 8**
> Don't Want to Miss a Thing: Susan on Assessment
>
> As you elicit the clients' narratives about their substance use, be sure to keep asking, "What else?" Until you are very sure you have exhausted all substance use pathways. Once, conducting an assessment, a client let Susan know they used alcohol and cannabis daily. She asked, "What else?" They talked about their use of cocaine at events like parties and live music shows. She asked, "What else?" They let her know that once a year, they would forage for opium poppy straws or pods, which they dried for use in teas, but this was seasonal and occasional. At that point, Susan thought she must have exhausted this clients' substance use. Months later, the client's addiction psychiatrist said she'd have to hold off on prescribing naltrexone to treat the client's alcohol use disorder due to his daily use of kratom, a partial opioid agonist. What?! His daily use of kratom? Susan realized she had missed a major aspect of the client's substance use that affected their relative risks. The lesson: Be sure to keep asking, "What else?"

It is important to understand the full picture of your clients' substance use, including the specific substances used (i.e., quantity, frequency, route of administration), substance-related harm, set (emotional, motivational, cultural reasons for use or nonuse as well as expectancies from use), and setting (physical, environmental, social, cultural).

The SIP is an easy-to-administer, psychometrically sound and universally applicable way to assess substance-related harm trajectories

Once this picture is obtained, it is important to engage the universal measure of harm reduction we use with all clients, the Short Inventory of Problems (SIP), which we introduced in Chapter 3 (see SIP-AD in Appendix 3).

- Introducing the SIP: "As we have discussed, this is harm reduction treatment, and my job as a harm reduction clinician is to support you in reduc-

ing your substance-related harm. One way we will check in to see we are on track and that I am doing my job right is to measure your experience of substance-related harm once a month using a measure called the Short Inventory of Problems or the SIP. How does that sound to you?" Answer any questions or concerns a client may have.
- Bring out the measure, turn it toward your client, and read off the instructions at the top, "I am going to read to you a number of events people sometimes experience in relation to their substance use. Please indicate how much each has happened to you in the past 30 days by telling me the appropriate number, where 0 = *never*, 1 = *once or a few times*, 2 = *once or twice a week*, and 3 = *daily or almost daily*."
- Leaving the questionnaire facing the client, read each prompt, repeating the time frame and the scale anchors every time. We find if we do not repeat these, people draw on events that happened longer than 30 days ago, or they have the tendency to rush to the "worst" response (e.g., "All threes!") without thinking about how often they have actually experienced each. That said, if a person continues to experience negative sequelae from events further in the past, that is ok to record, depending on the item. If a person asks you how to interpret the items, encourage them to be autonomous in their process. For example, "Whatever that means to you is the right answer." We really want to center clients' own personal responses to each.

Assessment Feedback. When the assessment stage is done, it is important to be nonjudgmental and compassionate in your delivery of feedback and summary of the assessment and to focus on specific examples and numbers they reported. Here are some examples of how feedback may be delivered using different measures:
- "As you remember, we are focused on reducing substance-related harm in harm reduction treatment."
- *Feedback regarding quantity and frequency:* "Looking at the questions we went through before [or that you completed with assessment person], it appears you are currently using xx on xx days a month. On a typical day, you said you use about xx grams of [substance]/drink xx drinks. On your heaviest day in the past month, you said you used xx/drank xx. Does that sound about right?" (If set and setting are particularly salient aspects of use or figure heavily into relative risks, you can also provide feedback on set and setting.)
- "You also said you have been experiencing some harm/problems/not-so-good things/negative side effects, such as... [Fill in specific examples from the SIP]. Did I get that down right?"
- *As applicable in your practice:* "In harm reduction, we also really care about how you are doing overall – not just about substance use. What other things would you like to measure that would help us decide how harm reduction treatment is working for you? For some clients, this has meant measuring specific harms, including alcohol-related seizures, blackouts, or overdoses."
- "What else would you like to measure that is important to you in your healing/recovery?" Be prepared to measure other aspects clients might be interested in as well, including other psychiatric symptoms (e.g., depression

Help demystify the numbers for clients and invite their input so they understand their own trajectories

or anxiety measures), biomarkers, or QoL measures (see Sections 3.3.2. through 3.3.4).
- Note: For an example of a conversation involving feedback on liver function tests, if you are administering them, please see Section 4.3.1.

Remember that after you introduce the feedback for one of the measures, elicit clients' responses to it: "Does that sound about right to you?" or "What does that number mean to you?" This will help you gauge if you are correct in your summary and what clients are doing with that information.

Client-Led Tracking. In Figure 10, you will find an example of a blank tracking progress grid on which you can help clients record substance-related harm as measured by the SIP (and as applicable, other outcomes of their choice) along the y-axis and changes over time along the x-axis. In our research studies, we have used a hardcopy version of this tracking grid, whereas in the clinic, data are entered into a spreadsheet program, graphed, and printed for clients. We now also have the measures and graphing built into our clinic EHR system.

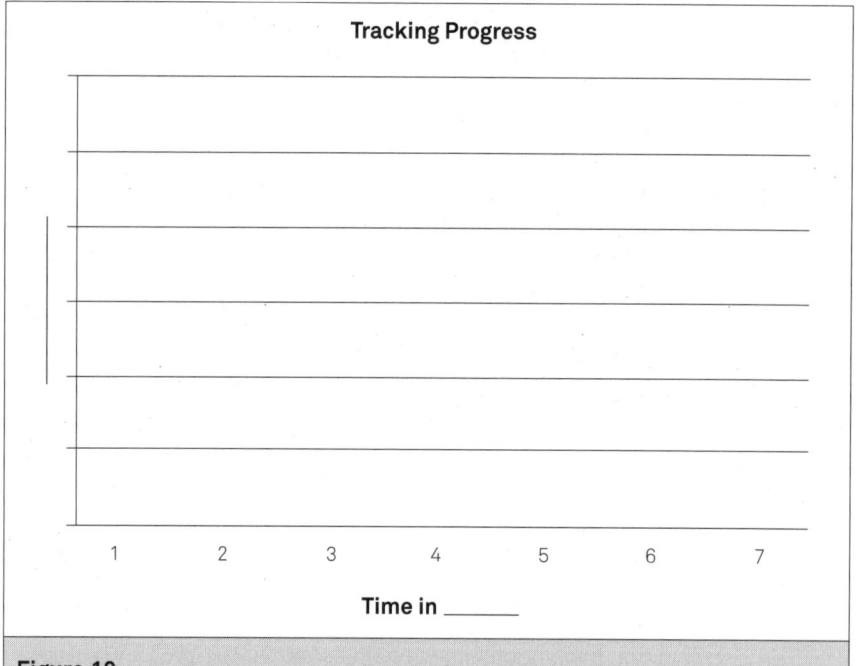

Figure 10
Tracking form example. This form is also available in Appendix 4 for personal/professional use.

You might say:
- "As I have mentioned, we are engaged in harm reduction treatment. Because my job is to help you reduce the harms you experience when you use substances, we will be tracking your scores on the SIP, which is a measure of substance-related harm, on this graph. That way, we can see how I'm doing in supporting you, and if we need to, we can change things up to better get you where you want to be."

- "Often, people find it helpful to track other outcomes – other measures of harm, substance use, mental health, or quality of life – over time so they can see how these things change and connect with each other. Which of these would you like to track over time?"
- "Great! Each [name timeframe here], we will be tracking these outcomes as one way to check in and see how things are going from [time to time]."
- "How does that sound?"

Depending on the treatment trajectory for clients, you can repeat this process of assessment, feedback, and tracking at each session or at regular intervals. The SIP is always tracked at monthly intervals, given its time frame; however, if needed, you can reduce the time frame of the SIP down to 2 weeks without changing the original measure. Always be sure to use the same timeframe, however, to ensure accurate reflection of overall experience of harm.

Establishing Client-Driven, Harm Reduction Goals

Some clients have goals in mind when they talk to a treatment professional. Others may have given this topic less thought. Still others are convinced that *you* believe the only legitimate goal is abstinence and might feel compelled to say what they think you would like to hear. This is why it is important to use simple, open-ended questions to elicit treatment goals that clients believe are reachable and desirable. Make this a fluid conversation in which you get to know the goals that are closest to your client's heart. Elicit and listen carefully to clients' own narratives and stories about what they want to see happen for themselves and why, and reinforce these goals.

Harm reduction goals are client-driven

You may elicit these goals by asking:
- "We will be meeting over the next [xx amount of time]. What would you like to see happen for yourself?"
- "Some people call this a goal, a vision or an intention." Be sensitive to and honor the client's preferred terminology around goals – those might be hopes, desires, visions, intention, prayers. Write them down under "What I want to make happen" (and replace terminology as needed) on the SHaRE form (see Figure 5 and Figure 6 as well as client handout in Figure 11 and Appendix 6).
- "What else?/What other goals are you interested in achieving for yourself?"
- As needed, ask further: "Do you foresee any barriers to achieving these goals?" If the client seems stuck with implementation, you can also ask, "What can I do to help you work toward that goal?"
- If clients rush to abstinence-based or use reduction goals, which might be a sign of premature treatment focus, remind them of the HaRT rationale: "Just as a reminder, in harm reduction treatment, I am not going to ask you to change your use in any way you don't want to. Instead, I am here to help you reduce your substance-related harm and improve your quality of life on your own terms. So, what do YOU want to see happen for yourself?"

In our work, clients have shared the fact that experiencing successes with goals that are affirmed and reinforced by clinicians is very important them. Thus, we want clients' goals – particularly those in the earlier sessions – to be achievable within the next week, to ensure this process builds

Goals must be of a nature and number that is achievable by the next session

> **What I want to make happen for myself**
>
> - Talk to case manager about voc counseling – Thurs 3pm (getting back to work)
>
> - _____

Figure 11
Harm reduction goals form that clients can take with them. This form is also available in Appendix 5 for personal/professional use. On the reverse side, we typically have a list of the safer-use strategies printed (see Appendix 1).

clients' self-efficacy and autonomy in reaching the goals they set for themselves. So, if clients mention larger goals that may be difficult to achieve right away (e.g., "getting back to work") – even if clients are enthusiastic about this goal – help them to break these goals down into more achievable pieces. You might say, "That's a great goal [affirmation]! It's also a big goal. What do you think is the first step in achieving that goal?"

You may then help clients visualize the stepwise nature of goal setting, using the visual aid in Figure 12. You can record the larger goal (e.g., "getting back to work") in the top step. Then, go back down to the bottom step, and ask the client to name the first step toward that larger goal that they can take in the next week. This stair-step model can be used from week to week to guide clients' incremental progress toward a larger goal. Again, it is *not* important in HaRT that clients achieve a certain goal in a certain way on a certain timeline. Instead, it is most important that this process helps to build clients' self-efficacy and autonomy around goal setting on their own recovery pathway.

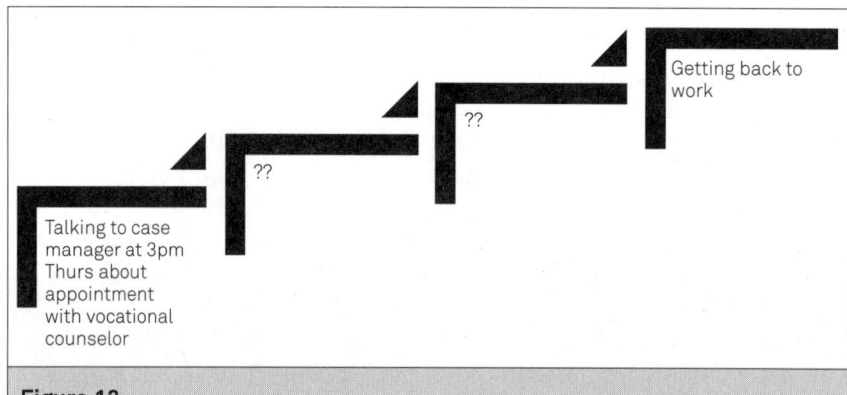

Figure 12
Stair-step approach to honing harm reduction goals.

Goals are recorded on the SHaRE form in our research studies (see Figure 5). In EHRs, we have simply created numbered lists of goals in our therapy notes with a header (e.g., "current week's goals"). If you have broken down larger goals into smaller goals for the following week, write in the smaller goal first at the numbered line. Then, in parentheses, write down the larger goal on the same line.

As you write down goals on the SHaRE form (see Figure 5) or in your numbered list, help clients copy the same onto the handout to take with them (see Figure 11 and Appendix 6). Then, close out this section by being affirming and reminding clients you will be checking in the next week about their goals. Goal setting and follow-up should be an ongoing, routine process that drives your sessions: "Thank you for sharing with me what you want to see happen! I have written it down in my records, and we have it here for you to take with you as well. That way, you can remind yourself about what you want to make happen for yourself this week. I look forward to checking in with you next week to see how things went!"

Introducing Safer-Use Strategies

Even if clients are not interested in reducing use or achieving abstinence, there are still things they can do to decrease the risk of harm they experience due to substance use. You can now introduce the safer-use strategies that best apply to their current substance use and goals (see Appendix 1) and engage clients in a discussion of the safer-use strategies that they may try out over the next few weeks.

Safer-use strategies can help clients make life-saving changes on their own terms and timelines

To introduce this discussion, we suggest showing the safer-use strategies to clients (see Figure 13 and Appendix 1 for all safer-use strategies pages).

Then, you can use the following step-by-step script to ensure positive uptake and avoid discord:
1. Explain the form overall: "I care about you and how you are doing, so I want to share with you some ways you can stay safer and healthier, even if you continue using [xx]."
2. Introduce one category of safer-use strategies at a time: "This first category represents things you can do to stay healthier without changing your use at all."
3. Provide one example strategy for each category that is relevant for your client based on your prior assessment: "This category includes eating before you use as a safer-use strategy."
4. Provide brief psychoeducational information as to why that example helps people stay safer/healthier: "This is important because if you sometimes forget to eat when you are using, your body won't have the nutrients it needs to power through and recover."
5. Repeat for the remaining two categories, like this:
    - "The second category includes ways to change the way in which you use to reduce your substance-related harm. An example here is not mixing uppers and downers. One of the risks is that uppers can – for a short time – cover up an overdose on downers like fentanyl. It also pulls your system in two different directions and stresses your heart."

Safer-use strategies are ways to stay healthier, change the manner of or reduce use on clients' own terms

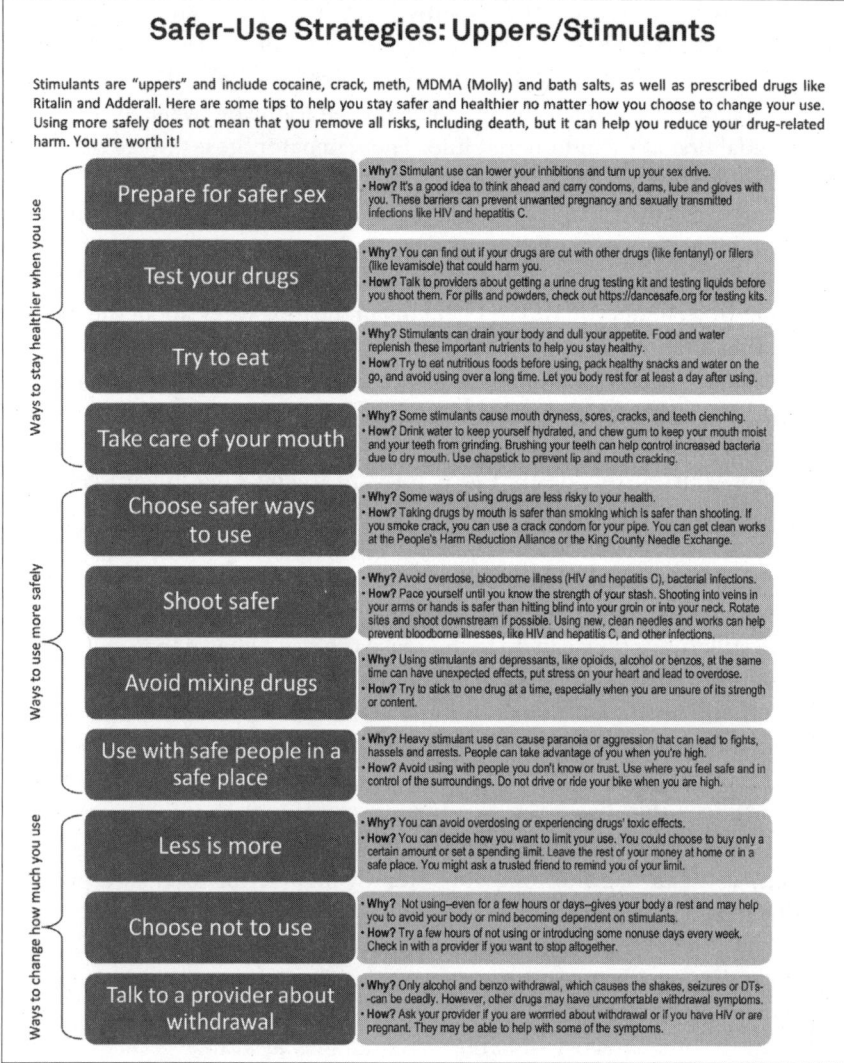

Figure 13
Safer-use strategies for stimulants. This form, as well as safer-use strategies for alcohol and depressants, are available in Appendix 1 for personal/professional use. Source: https://depts.washington.edu/harrtlab/wordpress/wp-content/uploads/2018/11/Safer-Use-Stimulants.pdf

- "Finally, you can change how much you use. For example, you can choose not to use in certain situations or at certain times. That gives your body a break and can keep you from needing the substance to function. [Note: If client is already physically dependent, add the following statement.] Be sure, however, you consider the importance of avoiding withdrawal. It can be life-threatening if you are self-withdrawing from alcohol or benzos. Withdrawal from other substances can be very unpleasant. We can discuss ways to avoid this happening to you."

6. Next, inquire if the client has ever tried any of the things on the list before to reduce the harm they experience while using substances ("Have you ever tried doing anything on this list before?").

7. If so, ask clients: "How did that go?" or "What was that like for you?" Most people have done some things on the list, so this affirms and honors what they are already doing to reduce their substance-related harm.
8. Support clients' self-efficacy by reinforcing and affirming the client's efforts to date, and provide the psychoeducational information to inform them about why that is safer. For example: "Sounds like a good choice! Avoiding mixing coke and fentanyl is a healthier decision because coke revs you up while fentanyl brings you down. As I mentioned, that can lead to accidental overdose and stress your body. Way to make a safer choice."
9. Ask what safer-use strategies they can try over the next week. Check or circle these for clients on the safer-use strategies form that best applies to their primary substances (see Appendix 1 for all safer-use strategy forms). Clients can also add their own tips.
10. Inform clients you will check in with them during the next meeting about their safer-use strategies to see how it worked out for them.
11. Clients should receive the safer-use strategies handout (see Appendix 1) with their harm reduction goals (see Appendix 5) recorded for them on the back for them to take with them.
    - Do not worry that you are enabling clients by talking about safer-use strategies. Our research shows that quite the opposite is true: You are likely helping to save their lives (see Box 19).
    - Never read off the entire form or go over every single strategy. That is too didactic and time-consuming. Also, do not just hand it to the client, because it would be hard to take it all in without the above orientation.
    - Again, after you introduce the safer-use strategies page(s), be sure to elicit what strategies clients have tried before and their narrative around those. This will ensure clients commit to safer use, on their terms and with greater intrinsic motivation.
    - If clients have already mentioned wanting to reduce their use or to use more safely as one of their goals, this can be pointed out on the list, and this goal can be explicitly reinforced as a step toward safer use.

> **Box 19**
> **Talking About Safer-Use Strategies Does Not Enable People to Use – It Enables People to Live**
>
> Some clinicians understandably have concerns about "enabling" clients to use if they talk about safer-use strategies. Fortunately, we have conducted research showing that HaRT, which does not require abstinence or use reduction and strives to help people reduce substance-related harm, is associated with *reduced use and reduced substance-related harm* (Collins, Clifasefi et al., 2019; Collins, Duncan et al., 2021). In fact, our most recent research study shows that people who committed to using safer-use strategies around staying healthier (not changing their use at all) when drinking had less alcohol-related harm over time (Alawadhi et al., 2023)! Thus, talking about safer use is does not harm clients, it help keep clients alive. And if clients are still alive, they can stay clinically connected and have ongoing chances to make positive behavior changes for themselves, their families, and their communities.

Wrapping Up

Thank clients for their time, and willingness and openness to talk to you. Let clients know that you value their feedback about the session. Ask them how they felt it went, and what you could do to improve the usefulness of these appointments. If they have suggestions, take these on board for future sessions. Be sure they have their copy of the safer-use strategies and goals. Schedule clients for their next appointment. Ask them if they have any further questions.

Follow-Up HaRT Sessions

The follow-up sessions include the following (three key components are bolded):
- Opening the session (2 minutes)
- **Reviewing substance use assessment and client-led tracking (5 minutes)**
- **Checking in about goals established in the prior session and establishing next set of goals (10 minutes)**
- **Checking in about safer substance use plan established in the prior session and establishing new plan (10 minutes)**
- Wrapping up (5 minutes)

Prior to this session, review clients' substance use assessment, previously stated goals, safer substance use plans, concerns, and/or questions. This will help you prepare for the session.

Follow-up sessions will likely take less time than the initial session. Leftover time can be used troubleshooting challenges and eliciting stories around and affirming positive changes. As HaRT moves further down the timeline, you can also introduce additional interventions, such as cognitive behavioral strategies, existential or humanistic psychotherapy, mindfulness or other psychotherapeutic tools, as long as they align with clients' goals and the HaRT mindset and heartset. You may also introduce new assessment and feedback tools when clients are facing new decisions about their use. When clients are introducing new substances or need to make decisions about use or other goals, using a decisional balance can be a helpful tool (i.e., helping clients write down and consider lists of pros and cons). The decisional balance allows you to assess the positive things clients like about their use as well as the not-so-good things. By acknowledging the whole picture, you can build a better therapeutic alliance, assess where a client is in their motivation for change, and understand what their substance use is "doing" for them. You can then creatively brainstorm how clients may achieve the positive things they like about their substance use while minimizing the harm.

Opening the Session

Greet clients, offer them light refreshments, and thank them for taking the time to talk to you. Remind them you are a harm reduction clinician, and they are doing HaRT, which is all about helping them reduce their substance-related harm and improve their QoL on their own terms and their own timeline. Remind them that you will not ask them to change their use in any way they do not want to. Briefly review the treatment course timeline so clients have clear expectations about upcoming visits as well as the day's agenda. Elicit any questions clients have.

Reviewing Substance Use Assessment and Tracking

Next, elicit a story about their substance use over the last xx time: "Tell me a little about how things have been going since we last met." If that general narrative does not include information about their substance use, ask a follow-up question like: "Tell me a little about how things have gone with your substance use" or "How has your substance use figured in [to whatever story they told you about]?" Be sure as you elicit this narrative, which will provide your assessment information, you engage in active listening and use your harm reduction strengths-based OARS.

Provide a summary statement of the clients' substance use assessment based on their responses to the narrative elicitation, questionnaires, and/or measures. It is important to be nonjudgmental and compassionate in doing so and to focus on specific examples and numbers they reported as you did in the initial session.

If this is a tracking day for the SIP, which is assessed once a month, this information is added to the tracking form and shown to the client so they can see how this fits into the larger picture. You or the client can add the day's data point to its respective position on the tracking chart. Practice ahead of time so you can feel confident about this process. If you do, they will. And remember that everyone is a scientist if given a chance. In fact, many clients have told us that having access to their data and being able to track it themselves is empowering and have cited it as one of the reasons they decided to make substantial changes in their substance use and other health-related behaviors.

If clients' substance use and/or side effects according to the SIP have decreased (see Figure 14), be sure they note that on the chart. Elicit a story from the client about how they were able to make those changes, how that went, and how they feel about it. This is affirming in and of itself, but also be sure to provide affirmation for the positive steps they are taking toward being safer and healthier.

Some clients might have a flat or worsening trajectory on a measure (see Figure 15). In that case, seek to affirm the positive. For example, affirm them for having come to the session – "That is a really huge step toward making a change!" – and for working toward other goals. Affirm them for other things that they have been doing positively.

Client-Driven Goals

Ask clients about their progress toward their goals. For example, "Last time we discussed your goals. You told me you were interested in getting back to work. For this week specifically, you had planned to talk to your case manager about getting connected with the vocational counselor. How did that go for you?"

Using open-ended questions and prompts, you can encourage clients to tell you about their experiences. Focus on eliciting a story and *not* simply asking about whether they achieved the goal or not. Additionally, verbally and enthusiastically affirm any positive steps they have taken toward achieving their goals. Record clients' progress toward or achievement of goals in the

---

Sidebar:

Elicit the story about clients' use so you better understand their driving narrative and the drug, set and setting

You can provide strengths-based affirmations, no matter what the clients' trajectories in tracking look like – even coming back to talk to you is celebrated

In assessing goals, elicit a story – Do not simply ask whether a goal was achieved or not

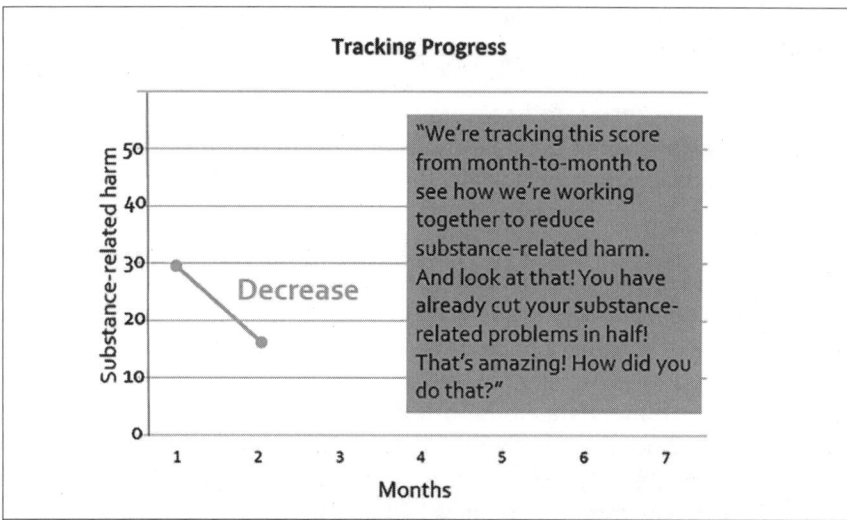

Figure 14
Tracking progress form and interpretation script if clients show relative improvement on the measure (e.g., Short Inventory of Problems for Alcohol and Drugs [SIP] Measuring Substance-Related Harm).

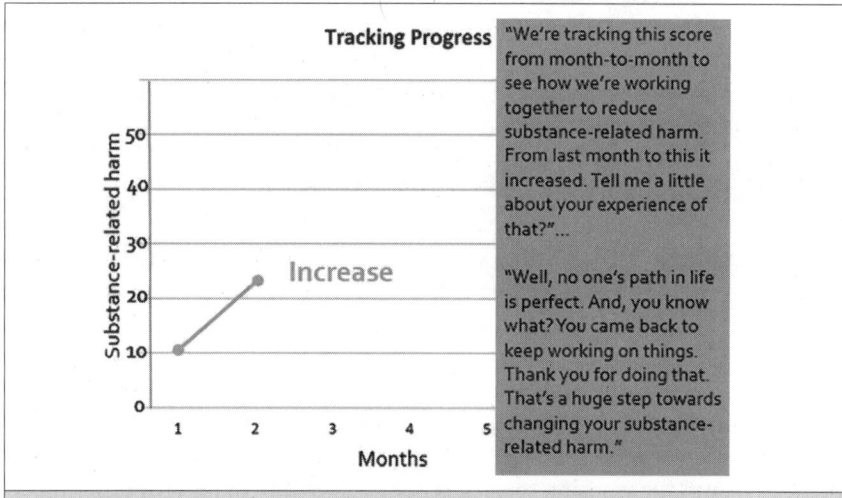

Figure 15
Tracking progress form and interpretation script if clients show flat or worsening trajectories on the measure (e.g., Short Inventory of Problems for Alcohol and Drugs [SIP] Measuring Substance-Related Harm).

appropriate place on the SHaRE form section for the previous visit, and add comments as necessary.

Next, using the dialogue suggested in the initial session, elicit and support additional goals for focus in the next [use appropriate time frame]. For example, you could say, "So, over the next week until we see each other again, what would you like to see happen for yourself?" Record these on both clients' new handout and on the SHaRE form. This can include continued work on a goal or renewal of the same goals.

Safer-Use Strategies
Check in about the safer-use strategies the client had committed to during the previous session. You can prompt them by saying,
- "Last time, you were going to avoid mixing cocaine and fentanyl. How did that go?"
- "Last time, you told me you wanted to try the a 'less is more' strategy. Specifically, you were going to try to stick to six regular beers instead of drinking four 211s each day. How did that go?"
- "Last time, you mentioned you would be sure to drink more water when using, by putting the water bottle on your nightstand. How did that go?"
- "Last time, you mentioned you were going to try to eat before using. How did that go?"

Again, be sure to *elicit a story* versus simply checking off whether they had engaged (or not) in safer-use strategies.

Record engagement in safer-use strategies on the SHaRE form for the previous visit. Then, refer clients to the safer-use strategies worksheet, and ask clients what safer-use strategies they would be interested in trying until the next session, using the suggested prompts provided in the initial session. Circle or check these so clients can see which ones they endorsed. These should also be recorded on the SHaRE form (or in the EHR) under "Client's Safer Substance Use Plan."

General Notes on Safer Use and Goals Assessment
If clients report having achieved their goals or safer substance use plans, be sure to reinforce that: "Congratulations on making this commitment and sticking to it! What was that like sticking to your goal [or safer substance use plan] this week/month?" or "What differences did you notice?"

If clients report not having achieved their goals or safer substance use plan, be sure to encourage them to try again using nonjudgmental and supportive language. You should be sure to convey warmth, compassion, and pragmatism, regardless of their response. You might say: "Change can occur in small steps. Even committing to this goal [or safer substance use plan] is another step towards reducing your harm. What do you think about trying toward this goal [or safer substance use plan] again for this next week [or month]?"

To elicit an account of any barriers encountered, you might say: "Ok, you tried [xx] over the past [xx], and it didn't work out quite the way you wanted it to. But you are back this week, so that is a huge step toward harm reduction. Good for you! What could help you to keep trying toward this goal this next week? What would you do differently this week to try again?"

You can also ask clients:
- "On a scale from 0 to 10, where 0 is not at all important, and 10 is very important, how important is this goal [or safer substance use plan] to you?"
- "On a scale from 0 to 10, how confident are you that you can achieve this goal [or safer substance use plan]?"

If this is a lower number, ask clients, "What would it take for you to move from a 3 to a 6?" And help them problem solve around this. "What can I do to help you achieve this goal [or safer substance use plan]?" If they are no longer interested in that goal or safer substance use plan, elicit new strategies that resonate more with them where they are currently at. That's ok, too!

Regardless of clients' outcomes, you should take this opportunity to provide affirmation for coming to the meeting: "The fact that you came in today shows your commitment to working towards your goals and safer substance use. That's great!"

Ask clients about any other efforts they have been making since you last saw them – maybe working with their case manager, going to support groups, or going to spiritual services. Be sure to reinforce those other, related efforts as well.

Wrapping Up

Thank clients for their time and openness in talking to you. Let clients know that you value their feedback about the session and that you would like to ask them how they felt it went and what you could do to improve the usefulness of these meetings. Be sure they have their copy of the safer substance use steps or goals. Schedule clients for their next follow-up appointment. Ask them if they have any further questions.

4.1.4 Auxiliary HaRT Components

Earlier, we provided information on how to implement the behavioral aspects of HaRT (see Section 4.1.3). In this section, we provide auxiliary HaRT components and scripts to help you integrate HaRT into more medicalized settings or with medication-assisted treatment. Please note, these are scripts based on specific study protocols, so they are not meant to be exhaustive resources but rather a starting point.

Providing Feedback on Biomarkers

In case you are working within a more medicalized setting, we provide a template for how to deliver feedback on biomarkers.

Feedback on Liver Function Tests

Biomarkers can enrich feedback and tracking with physical indications of substance-related harm and subsequent harm reduction

In this first case, we provide a template for feedback on liver function tests (LFTs) in the context of AUD. It is important to first give clients some context for what the biomarkers mean generally. For example: "Your liver is amazing! It does so much for your body and to maintain your health. It produces energy your body needs, and it filters and neutralizes impurities and poisons in your bloodstream. It is especially important to monitor how the liver is doing when you drink, because alcohol damages the liver by causing inflammation. If this inflammation becomes chronic, it causes liver scarring and, in some cases, it causes liver cells to die. This is called cirrhosis. Even before people develop cirrhosis, we can see the physical changes in the liver as a leakage of chemicals into the blood. When this happens, we see high values on these blood tests."

You might ask at this point, "Have you heard this before?" or "Does this make sense?" to involve clients in the discussion and confirm their comprehension.

If LFTs are within normal ranges, you might say: Our lab tests indicate that your LFTs are within the normal range. This is not a guarantee that you have no liver damage at all, but it indicates your liver is functioning as expected. So yay! This is also a good sign, because you can probably reduce your experience of alcohol problems before it does permanent damage. We will talk about some ways you might be able to do this later on [revisit in your discussion of safer-use strategies].

If liver function tests are above the *upper limit of normal* (ULN): "Our lab tests indicate that your LFTs are above the normal range, which means that your liver is not functioning normally and may already have some physical damage. This damage can be caused by use of alcohol and/or other drugs and certain illnesses like hepatitis. Fortunately, you may be able to reduce some of the harm done to your liver. We will talk about some ways you might be able to do this later on [revisit this topic in your discussion of safer-use strategies]."

Feedback on Smoking-Related Biomarkers

In our research studies, we have used both hand-held carbon monoxide and spirometry equipment to measure and provide feedback for clients (see Chapter 3 for more information about these devices).

For carbon monoxide measurement, you might say: "We will measure how much carbon monoxide – which is one of the deadly chemicals in car exhaust – you are taking in when you breathe in cigarette smoke. This is important, because when you breathe, your lungs usually are feeding your red blood cells with oxygen. Your red blood cells then carry this oxygen all through your body to be sure your cells can breathe – all the way out to your organs and your fingers and toes. If you are breathing in smoke instead of pure oxygen, your lungs feed your red blood cells car exhaust instead of oxygen and carry that throughout your body. This starts to suffocate your cells. This means certain parts of your body might not work as well anymore because they aren't getting enough oxygen. So, we measure this because, if people reduce their smoking, they reduce the carbon monoxide they take in. That's one thing we can measure for you to track your progress over time."

Then, you report to them the CO level they had on the handheld device discussed in Section 3.3.3 (see Figure 16). You can show them the chart indicating what the various CO levels mean and get their thoughts on that: "What do you think of that?"

For *spirometry measurement*, you might note, "We can measure how well people's lungs are functioning. Smoking impacts that, too, because all the chemicals in cigarette smoke cause inflammation in the lungs. Over time, if these cells are continually inflamed, they can die. That makes people's lungs work less well, and this can lead to lung diseases like chronic obstructive pulmonary disease or COPD. So, we measure this because, if people reduce their smoking, they can find that – over time – their lungs feel like they are working better. That's another thing we can measure for you to track your progress over time."

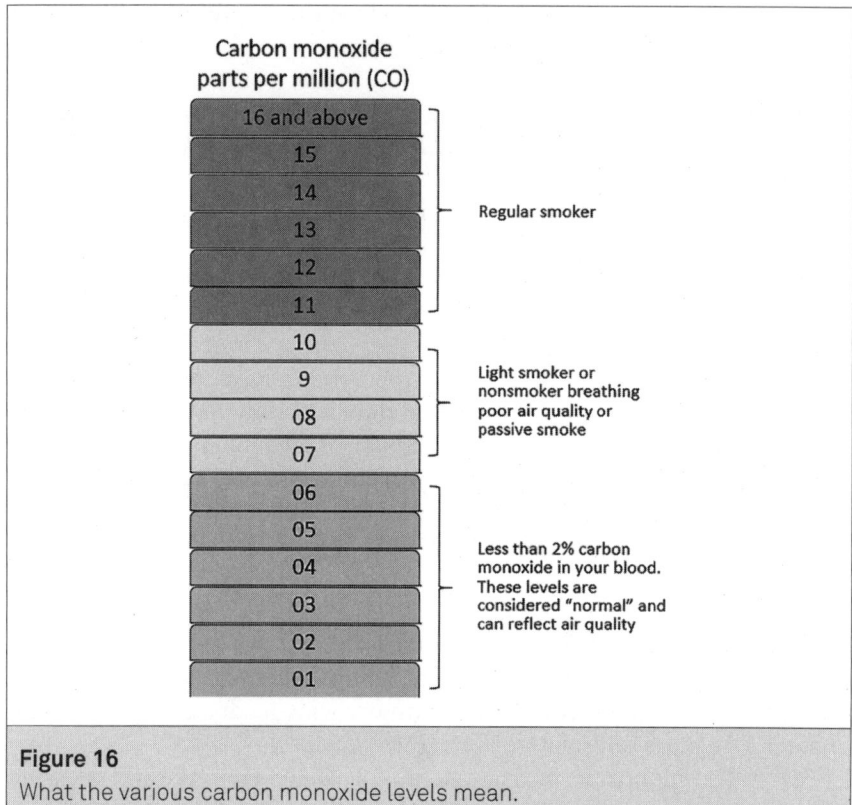

Figure 16
What the various carbon monoxide levels mean.

Then, you report to them their percentage lung function (FEV1%) and their estimated lung age using the data on the Feedback of Assessment form. Check in with them: "What do you think of that?" and "What does that mean to you?"

Next Steps

Generally, you will then tie feedback on the biomarkers into the rationale for the treatment and the components of the session. You might say: "These symptoms that bother you and some of the things you don't like as much about your [type of substance use] are what we are trying to focus on in this session – maybe improving your [liver health, lung health], like we just measured. We can track that over time. But know that I will not be asking you to change your [type of substance use] in any way that you don't want to. What I will do is work with you to figure out what you would like to get out of our time together and to help support you in achieving those goals you have. I also want to help you lessen your experience of substance-related harm and help you figure out ways you can use more safely. How does that sound?"

This is typically a good segue into any of the other HaRT components: comparing trajectories in the tracking part of the treatment, eliciting harm reduction goals, and/or discussing safer-use strategies.

Pharmacological Adjuncts

If you are using pharmacological adjuncts or medications for SUD, we have a few additional suggestions and example scripts to share from our study combining the behavioral HaRT described above with extended-release naltrexone (XR-NTX) in treating AUD (Collins, Duncan, et al., 2021; Collins, Duncan, et al., 2015). Please note that your exact approach to assessment and manner of pharmacobehavioral treatment integration will depend on the client, the substances they use and mode of use, your assessments, your setting, your professional identity and that of your team, and the specific medications or pharmacological adjuncts used. If you are not a medical professional yourself, how you proceed should be tailored accordingly in conjunction with medical consultation.

> Behavioral HaRT components can be interwoven into the rationale for harm reduction medications and pharmacological adjuncts

Integrating Medication Management and Behavioral HaRT Approaches

To the extent possible, we suggest finding ways to integrate the medical and behavioral assessments and treatment components in a way that minimizes barriers to accessing service (e.g., deliver them in the same appointments, provide access in community-based settings). In our research, we have fully integrated these two aspects of the treatment with much success, and suggest consulting guides on integrated behavioral health approaches for ways to integrate care and teams for substance use treatment (Collins, Duncan, et al., 2016).

Administering a Medical Assessment

In addition to the assessment strategies offered in Chapter 3, you should (or should be working with medical professionals to) take vital signs, assess medical history, conduct a physical, take any necessary blood and urine samples, and complete a medication reconciliation to rule out any interaction effects or manage them responsibly. Regular appointments with physicians and nurses are important to ensuring the safety and efficacy of medication-assisted treatment; however, ensure that appointments are as low-barrier as possible to bolster client engagement and maximize their autonomy.

Explaining How Pharmacological Adjuncts Can Help

We recommend introducing the medication as integrated with the behavioral HaRT and showing how combining the medication and behavioral aspects of the treatment can synergistically support clients in achieving their goals and safer use. We specifically suggest tying feedback from assessment, goals, and safer use, to the medication. Here are example scripts illustrating this step from our study on HaRT plus XR-NTX: "The side effects of alcohol you told us about last week indicate that your [mind, body or both] need alcohol to function normally. For example, you mentioned xx [provide an example from the assessment here, such as "you mentioned needing to drink in the morning to stop the shakes"]. Have you ever heard this before [or has your doctor ever told you this before]?"

Wait for the participant's response and weave what they say into your definition, if on target. It is also important to tie this feedback into the treatment rationale and the components of the session. You might say: "These symptoms that bother you and some of the things you don't like as much about your alcohol use are what we are trying to focus on in this session. I will not be asking you to change your drinking in any way that you don't want to. What I do want to do is work with you to figure out what you would like to see happen for yourself, and to work with you to be sure any medications I prescribe can help you achieve that specific goal. We can also find ways that medications might help you decrease the harm you experience when you use [or to help you be safer when you use]. How does that sound?"

You will then want to introduce the medication(s) that might be helpful (in this case XR-NTX), explain how it works and how it might be compatible with and help them achieve their goals. Remember to weave in participants' stated goals throughout your interview with them. You might start with: "Now we have some goals that you are working toward, such as [reiterate participants' stated goals]. I would like to tell you a little bit about how [this specific medication/adjunct] might help you achieve your goals."

To tailor this, focus on what clients wanted to achieve in their stated goals. For example, according to scientific studies, XR-NTX can:

- Reduce cravings and desire to drink
- Help people reduce heavier drinking
- Enhance people's QoL by improving their
  - Mental health functioning
  - Social functioning
  - Physical functioning
- Can help people maintain abstinence

It is important to reiterate that medications will not resolve all of the not-so-good things about their substance use. However, depending on the medication and the substance clients are using, medications might give them more confidence about reaching their goals and support them in safer use.

Demystify the Medication's Mechanism of Action, Risks, and Benefits

It is empowering for clients to have information about the treatments and to be able to ask questions about them. To start this conversation, ask participants what they may already know about the medication, using open-ended questions. Affirm their asking questions. If necessary, clear up any myths (see Box 20 for an example) or misinformation participants may have, gently and asking permission. It is important to inform participants about the medication and its potential benefits and risks, in a way that is transparent and neither fear-inducing nor glossing over. Also, explain the mechanism of action, using figures and simple language. An example we used for our study with XR-NTX is shown in Figure 17.

Box 20
Need To Differentiate Among Medications and Debunk Myths

In the case of extended-release naltrexone, you may need to distinguish it from disulfiram (Antabuse). Most people have heard that disulfiram (Antabuse) makes people violently sick when combined with alcohol. They may confuse disufiram with naltrexone. Participants may thus have concerns about taking medications for treating alcohol use disorder.

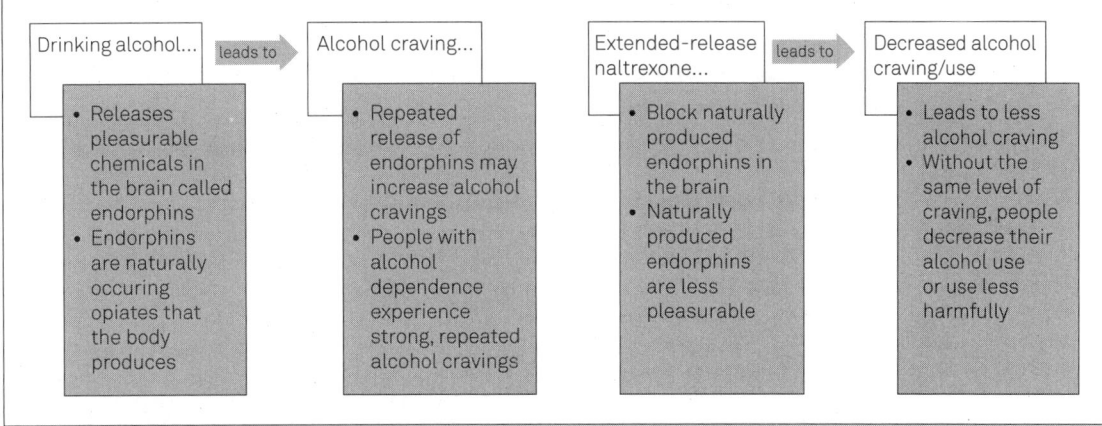

Figure 17
Extended-Release Naltrexone (XR-NTX) proposed mechanism of action. Adapted from Collins et al., 2021 (p. 49 in the supplementary appendix).

Explain Dosing

Help clients understand the menu of options of medications and dosing. In the case of our research on XR-NTX, there was only one formulation, so we informed participants that they would receive one, 380-mg injection of either placebo or XR-NTX into their gluteal (buttocks) muscle once a month for the next 3 months. XR-NTX is an extended-release formulation, so we let them know it works for 30 days before they need to get the next shot and that coming back for regular appointments would keep a regular level in their bloodstream to ensure the most consistent benefit. It is important to note that it may take a certain amount of time until they notice medications are working.

Being Transparent About Side Effects and Preparing Clients to Manage Them

It is also important to discuss potential side effects, while debunking any myths about side effects that participants may be concerned about. In Box 21, you find an example from our research on XR-NTX and HaRT.

Help prepare participants to manage side effects, as necessary. Regarding XR-NTX, we would tell clients:

- You can manage the most common side effects, nausea, stomach problems and headaches, by taking Pepto-Bismol® or over-the-counter pain reliever according to instructions.
- If you experience more serious symptoms, you should inform your provider immediately by calling the number listed here. On the phone, we will talk to you about your symptoms, advise on next steps, and arrange for you to be checked by a medical professional as soon as possible.
- With your permission, we may contact your case manager or primary care physician (PCP) to explain the situation and get you the proper follow-up care. Further, if we learn information during the study about conditions that pose immediate danger to your health and safety if you participate,

we will share this information with you, and if necessary, agency staff or your PCP to ensure your health and safety are protected.
- In case of emergency, please contact 911 as well as your case manager or health-care provider.

> **Box 21**
> **XR-NTX Side Effects and Potential Interaction Effects**
>
> - Extended-release naltrexone (XR-NTX) is not addictive. You can stop it anytime without experiencing withdrawal symptoms.
> - Side effects of XR-NTX may include decreased appetite, nausea, vomiting, upper abdominal pain, headache, back pain, dizziness, fatigue, irritation or itching at the injection site. Very rare symptoms have been reported such as pneumonia, depression, and suicidality. We will ask you questions about these symptoms at each meeting.
> - Primarily nausea, headache, and injection site reactions have caused about 9% (of 900 in controlled studies) of people to stop taking the medication.
> - At very high doses, the oral form of this medication has led to liver toxicity. This has not been the case with XR-NTX. However, this is the reason we monitor your liver functioning, because it gets broken down in your liver.
> - If you choose to drink, XR-NTX will not make you sick. However, it may cause you to feel fewer positive effects of alcohol the more you drink.
> - XR-NTX does not have psychological effects. It will not make you feel "high" or "down."
> - Interaction effects with other medications
> - You should *not* be given XR-NTX if you use opiates. It will block the effects of opiates in a way that can lead to opioid withdrawal or may lead you to overdose. Please let me know if you are taking opiates for whatever reason.
> - You should wear your ID tag and carry your emergency card with you, so doctors know that you are taking XR-NTX. This will help them arrange your pain management in case of an emergency.
> - XR-NTX does not interact with other commonly prescribed medications besides opiates.
> - Women in childbearing years must use effective birth control while on XR-NTX. The effects of XR-NTX on pregnancy have not been systematically studied in humans. If you become pregnant during the study, we will discontinue the medication.
> - I know this is a lot of information and some if it may seem scary. But each time we meet, I will ask you about side effects you may be experiencing to ensure your safety. Your safety, health, and well-being are the most important things for us.

4.2 HaRT Efficacy and Prognosis

4.2.1 Behavioral Harm Reduction Treatment for AUD

Over a 15-year period, we have used a multiphase community-based participatory research approach (Collins et al., 2018), to better understand the needs of the communities we work with (Clifasefi et al., 2016; Collins, Clifasefi, Andrasik, et al., 2012; Collins, Clifasefi, Dana, et al., 2012; Larimer et al., 2009; Stahl et al., 2016), and later, to develop, evaluate, and implement the HaRT approach more specifically (Clifasefi et al., 2016; Collins, Jones, et al., 2016). Most relevant to HaRT development, we conducted interviews with 50 people with lived experience of homelessness, AUD, and polysubstance, use to understand community perspectives on existing abstinence-based treatment and the community's vision for redesigning treatment to be more relevant, acceptable, desirable, and effective (Collins, Jones, et al., 2016). The findings indicated a lack of interest in existing abstinence-based approaches, which were considered to be institutionally oppressive, overly focused on abstinence, physically removed from their community, and mismatched to their own experiences and larger life context (Collins, Jones, et al., 2016). Instead, participants preferred client-driven, community-based, nonjudgmental, non-abstinence-based approaches that emphasize engagement in meaningful activities, personal goal setting, and discussions of safer-use strategies. These findings echoed those of other qualitative studies regarding preferences on programming content and treatment goals (Collins, Clifasefi, Dana, et al., 2012; Collins et al., 2015; Crabtree et al., 2018; Lee & Petersen, 2009).

Based on these stated preferences, researchers worked together with staff, management, and clients at community-based nonprofits to codevelop HaRT, among other interventions (Collins et al., 2018). HaRT was then administered in community-based settings and later in clinical settings in a randomized controlled trial involving non-treatment-seeking people who were experiencing homelessness and AUD, and who were polysubstance users (N = 168; Collins, Clifasefi, et al., 2019). Findings showed strong participant engagement. Among the 184 non-treatment seekers who were screened for participation in the initial randomized controlled trial, 99% consented, and 98% attended the baseline assessment. In keeping with the low-barrier, harm reduction approach, inclusion and exclusion criteria were minimal; thus, 92% of people who completed the screening and baseline assessment were included in the trial. Participants (N = 168) were randomized to receive the HaRT or simply their services as usual in their respective settings, which included a variety of services to help clients meet basic needs (e.g., emergency shelter, food provision, case management). At the final, 3-month follow-up, 74% of participants completed data collection. The vast majority (92%) of HaRT participants reported a positive treatment experience, whereas 8% had mixed or neutral perceptions of HaRT. No participants reported a negative perception of HaRT.

HaRT participants showed clinically meaningful reductions in peak alcohol quantity (–66%), alcohol-related harm (–71%), and number of AUD symptoms (–63%) across the 3-month study period, which translated into statistically significant differences between the HaRT and services-as-usual control conditions. Despite the fact that abstinence is not a priority or stated goal in harm reduction, HaRT participants evinced significantly fewer positive alcohol biomarker tests (–20%) over the course of the study compared with control participants (+19%; Collins, Clifasefi, et al., 2019).

4.2.2 Combined Pharmacotherapy and Behavioral Treatment

Extending the behavioral HaRT approach to the medication-assisted treatment context, we also conducted a successful pilot ($N = 31$; Collins, Duncan, et al., 2015) and, later, a randomized controlled trial (Collins et al., 2021) to test the efficacy of combining pharmacotherapy (i.e., XR-NTX) and HaRT for people experiencing homelessness, AUD and polysubstance use (80%). Participants were 308 adults experiencing homelessness and AUD who were receiving shelter and drop-in services at one of three community-based, nonprofit agencies in downtown Seattle, WA. Participants were randomized to one of four treatment arms: (a) behavioral harm reduction treatment for AUD framed for medical providers working in community-based service provision (HaRT) plus XR-NTX, (b) HaRT plus placebo injections, (c) HaRT only, and (d) supportive services treatment as usual (TAU) at their community-based setting.

Of those approached, nearly all (97%) were interested in participation, and over three fourths of participants in the HaRT + XR-NTX arm attended the final, Week 12 treatment session (Collins et al., 2021). Participants' stated goals focused on increasing meeting basic needs (27%), changing alcohol use (26%), enhancing QoL (21%), and improving health (16%), among others (10%); only 4% of participants' stated goals were to attain or maintain abstinence from alcohol (Fentress et al., 2021).

Compared with services as usual, the HaRT + XR-NTX arm evinced significant, baseline-to-posttreatment improvements across five of six outcomes: peak alcohol quantity, alcohol frequency, alcohol-related harm, alcohol biomarker tests, and physical health-related quality of life (HR-QoL). After treatment discontinuation at 12 weeks, improvements were maintained through the 36-week follow-up. Participants receiving HaRT + placebo and HaRT alone showed improvements across three of six outcomes compared with TAU (Collins et al., 2021). Despite the fact that HaRT was focused on reducing alcohol-related harm, a secondary analysis indicated that HaRT led to a reduction in frequency of cannabis and polysubstance use over the treatment course. There were no increases in use of any other substances over the treatment course (Mostofi & Collins, in press). Taken together, our findings to date have indicated that, compared with services as usual, combining HaRT and XR-NTX resulted in decreased substance use and alcohol-related harm, and improved physical HR-QoL for people experiencing homelessness, severe AUD, and polysubstance use.

4.3 Problems in Carrying Out the Approaches

It is important to acknowledge the challenges in practicing harm reduction in the US

Despite evidence indicating its positive effects for individuals, their communities, and society at large, it continues to be challenging to engage in harm reduction practices of all kinds in a world that still wants to blame and shame people who use substances, under the guise of "tough love." At a recent opioid overdose prevention taskforce meeting, one harm reduction advocate sighed heavily as she acknowledged that our collective work in harm reduction advocacy continues to be a perennial "lightening-rod issue."

There is no place where this is truer than in the treatment realm. Over the past 15 years, we have repeatedly had colleagues – some who even position themselves as advocates – pull us aside to correct us that we "should not explicitly say 'harm reduction'" in our talks, our grant applications, and our treatment resources. We have been told it is "too controversial." Recently, we were instructed via email by a senior administrator-level physician working in a methadone clinic that the term "harm reduction" has no place in treatment. We "should just call it 'client-centered care.'" In the past, we were told by senior-level administrators to rename our center because "harm reduction sounds so negative." We have also had people tell us they are practicing "harm reduction" in one breath, as they attempt to persuade clients to get sober in the next. "But, deep down, don't we really all want our clients to get sober?" pressed one highly esteemed colleague in the substance use treatment field after a talk.

We spend too much of our precious time parsing these terms, sanitizing our efforts for funding, and pushing against resistant systems for the inclusion and legitimization of harm reduction research and treatment services. Encumbered with those tasks, community members are dying at ever higher rates of alcohol-related liver disease and opioid overdose, most recently spurred on by a global pandemic that further isolated people who use substances and made in-person services more challenging to obtain and engage with. Most treatment agencies in the US have no harm reduction counseling or treatment services in their portfolio and are unaware of, or are resistant to, its adoption. Fortunately, we also conduct a lot of trainings in which providers, counselors, case managers, and social workers express deep gratitude for harm reduction and for HaRT. They finally have an evidence-based way to meet their clients where they are at, to help them stay safer and healthier, whether or not they are ready, willing, or able to stop using.

Of course, there are other systems pressures that hinder our efforts in harm reduction treatment and service provision. We have spent years working to debunk the unsubstantiated "enabling hypothesis," or concerns that harm reduction and non-abstinence-based approaches reinforce substance use or hinder recovery. Fortunately, the past few decades have provided extensive research to counter this unsupported assumption. We hope this work, as assembled in Sections 1.3 and 4.2, will provide you with the scientific information you need to spur important and informed discussions with your clients, colleagues, funders, and administrators.

The "enabling hypothesis" has been debunked by harm reduction research

Because of the debunked and yet widely believed enabling hypothesis, some family members and friends are concerned about harm reduction approaches. Our colleagues, the founders of the Harm Reduction Therapy Center, Patt Denning, PhD, and Jeannie Little, LCSW, have done excellent work in this area that we regularly recommend to friends and families of our clients (Denning, 2010; Denning & Little, 2017).

Based on this groundbreaking work, we often host family members in sessions when requested by clients to help provide an introduction to HaRT and help them forge boundaries they feel good about with their loved ones. Specifically, we encourage family and friends to consider what harm reduc-

We work with families and friends to create healthy boundaries to support harm reduction for all

tion looks like for them; we suggest they list the secondary harms they experience and distinguish between true harms and annoyances or hurts that may be negotiable or let go of. We ask them to also list the values they hold most dear. Then, we ask them to think of ways they can set boundaries in accordance with their values to manage or avoid the true harms they are experiencing due to their loved one's substance use. Instead of enabling, families feel empowered.

4.4 Diversity Issues

HaRT was co-developed with a diverse group of people with lived experience of social marginalization and SUD

As noted throughout this book, we used a community-based participatory research method to cocreate HaRT with people who use substances and come from diverse racial, ethnic, and cultural backgrounds, many of whom had lived experience of homelessness. We have worked with community-based agencies that are deeply embedded in the communities they provide services to, and have implemented the HaRT in community spaces as well as in clinics and hospital settings. Data currently being prepared for publication indicate that positive HaRT effects are not significantly different by race, ethnicity, and sex assigned at birth in people experiencing homelessness (Goldstein et al., 2023).

We acknowledge the limitations of Eurocentric, psychotherapeutic framework in which HaRT was developed

That said, HaRT might not meet all people where they are at. HaRT is conceptualized within a Western, Eurocentric psychotherapeutic model of care, which carries its own problematic history. First, psychotherapy has often been treated as if it can be applied universally – in research and in clinical practice – and does not need to be moderated by cultural humility or culturally specific knowledge (Sue, 2003). This accepted understanding of psychotherapy as a universally helpful construct has created biases in both the evidence base for, and application of, psychotherapeutic methods. Beyond psychotherapy, the field of psychology more broadly has only begun to grapple with its longtime collusion with eugenics and its deeply problematic applications of models of racial and cultural inferiority, pathology, and "cultural deprivation" (Leong & Park, 2016). In the field of substance use, White colonizers were largely responsible for introducing alcoholic beverages to Indigenous populations in the US, and yet White-dominated, Eurocentric health professions have used racist tropes to characterize substance use in Communities of Color (Duran, 1996). For hundreds of years, people who use substances were often vilified, criminalized, incarcerated, and/or institutionalized, and this practice has disproportionately affected Communities of Color and other minoritized and marginalized people (Collins, 2016), and the larger impacts of these pressures have been acknowledged in more recent years (e.g., https://www.apa.org/about/policy/dismantling-systemic-racism).

Studies addressing substance use treatment that have been conducted with Communities of Color have highlighted providers' and clients' concerns about the cultural acceptability of highly directive, Eurocentric approaches, such as cognitive behavior therapy and 12-step programming (Legha et al., 2014; Novins et al., 2011; Novins et al., 2016; Venner et al., 2012). Marginalized communities have pointed out the negative effects of power hierarchies, institutionalization, and punitive treatment when people are not ready, willing, or able to engage with abstinence-based approaches (Collins, Clifasefi, Dana, et al., 2012; Collins, Jones, et al., 2016). HaRT addresses some of these concerns given its community-based codesign, emphasis on advocacy, client-driven (vs. provider-driven) goal setting and centering client perceptions of QoL, but again, it utilizes a Western psychotherapeutic model.

> HaRT clinicians are called to be culturally humble and ensure clients receive culturally aligned treatment

There is a growing call to honor community-driven perspectives and engage more culturally appropriate healing and recovery pathways. Additionally, clinicians and researchers have begun to call for cocreation of community-based recovery programs that address historical trauma and bolster existing sources of strengths and resilience within the community (Ledesma, 2007). Naturally occurring strengths-based approaches in communities include storytelling about survival, building supportive social networks, and practicing cultural traditions (Kahn et al., 2016; Reinschmidt et al., 2016).

To this end, many are working with community members and community-based partners to bring research resources to the cocreation of more culturally appropriate harm reduction approaches (Dickerson et al., 2016; Nelson et al., 2022; Venner et al., 2018). However, as Western-trained harm reduction clinicians, and particularly when we do not identify as part of the community we are trying to serve, we must be culturally humble and take direction from the community. We must support communities in finding their own harm reduction pathways, support existing community sources of healing, and be respectful of the teachings so we are careful not to appropriate cultural practices that are not our own.

We also acknowledge and appreciate movements calling for the abolition of Western, Eurocentric counseling fields altogether, particularly in serving minoritized and marginalized populations (Toronto Abolition Convergence, 2020). These movements have led us to more actively interrogate our practices, evaluate our mistakes and the harm they cause, and learn more about abolition. We are grateful for our colleagues, friends, family, and community who have graciously noted our mistakes, allowed us to learn and become better allies and sometimes even accomplices in this work. Likewise, we encourage you, the reader, to find out more about your local community efforts in harm reduction and healing and support them through donations, volunteering, and culturally humble advocacy.

5

Afterword

Our dear friend and colleague, Mr. Joey Stanton, whom we cite throughout this book, was a harm reduction activist and advocate in his community. He was to be the third author of this book, but he died before we got started, at the beginning of the pandemic when our worlds were turned upside down, and we were separated by physical distancing and great loss. Years after his death, we regularly ask ourselves, "What would Joey do?" So, it seems most fitting to end this book reflecting on his words.

During a Grand Rounds talk we gave together at the University of Washington – Harborview Medical Center in June 2018, Susan asked Joey to "close us out." He did so with a plea to clinicians who, in Washington State, often have a "policy" of turning away people who are intoxicated from clinical appointments:

> It's all about power. When you start using power to try to help people, that's when it gets really messed up because I don't, I won't trust you. I didn't trust you. I'm not going to trust you. And I think a lot of people feel that way that are scared that [are saying], "I want to fucking die. I want to die." I wasn't saying that out loud, but that's what my actions were doing over and over and over and over again, and I couldn't figure it out. Now, I've learned that it's what I put in my body, but that, again, is my decision. It has nothing to do with your goddamn morals. That has to do with my decision to do what I want to.
>
> Harm reduction – if you're really serious about it – question policy. ... The next time you find yourself saying, "I can't do that because it is against policy," then start asking, "*Why* is that policy? What would work better?" Maybe [clinicians] can see people that are – oh God forbid – under the influence. Maybe we can see people who are substance users.

Typical Joey, he then laughed and said, "So, anyway, it's been fun, guys," to great applause from the gathered clinicians, counselors, and other professionals in the packed room.

For our part, we see you. We love you. The journey towards harm reduction is so many things. And, yes, it's been fun.

6

Case Vignettes

Ms. D.

Ms. D. was a 45-year-old, cisgender, heterosexual, urban Indigenous woman who had been chronically homeless for about 15 years before moving into a single-site Housing First program (i.e., low-barrier, permanent supportive housing). Ms. D. presented for and consented to a 3-month course of harm reduction counseling paired with XR-NTX in the context of a research study.

Separated from her family for many years, Ms. D. had strong ties to an adopted "street family" and a long-term, devoted partner who lived in the same Housing First program. Ms. D. had a long history of injection heroin use, through which she had contracted hepatitis C, which she reported had subsequently spontaneously resolved. She also had a history of daily alcohol use and had experienced multiple bouts of alcoholic hepatitis. In the 30 days prior to her initial assessment, Ms. D. reported daily smoking (roll-your-own tobacco cigarettes) and alcohol use. She also reported using cannabis (smoking) on 12 days, crack cocaine (smoking) on 3 days, and heroin (injecting) once.

Ms. D. was interested in participation but reported being wary of being told what to do by study staff. Together with her harm reduction clinician, an Indigenous addiction psychiatrist, she engaged in the HaRT + pharmacological support protocol outlined in this book. She attended three initial, weekly appointments, and then two additional monthly appointments during which she was assessed for substance use and substance-related harm and tracked these findings together with the harm reduction clinician, developed harm reduction goals and her progress towards them, and discussed safer-use strategies.

Ms. D.'s goals initially centered around reducing negative side effects of substance use and improving cognitive function. Later, she reported goals around improving her activities of daily living, particularly wanting to eat more as she began drinking less. Her harm reduction clinician notably engaged her around discussions of cooking and provided her with requested recipes to help her reconnect with a meaningful activity and to encourage eating as a safer-use strategy.

Although Ms. D. never expressed explicit interest in reducing her drinking or other drug use, by the end of the 3-month treatment period, she reported reducing days of cigarette smoking by one third (20/30 days), reducing her daily alcohol consumption by 26% and heaviest day of alcohol consumption by half, maintaining her crack consumption, and reporting no heroin use.

About 9 months after that study ended, our study team learned from housing staff she was in the hospital with another bout of alcoholic hepatitis.

The addiction psychiatrist who had worked with her during the study and I (Susan E. Collins) visited her in the hospital. She and the addiction psychiatrist initially engaged in the banter they often shared, as they had great rapport. Suddenly, he became very serious. He said, "Ms. D., I really care about you. And if you don't stop drinking, you're going to die."

At that point she fell silent and turned away to look out the window. The addiction psychiatrist and I exchanged glances. I raised my voice, saying to the addiction psychiatrist, "Ok, Dad, back off!" Ms. D. turned back to us, and half-smiling, rejoined, "Yeah, Dad!" I continued, "It's true, Ms. D. We care about you a lot, and we don't want to see you die. But really, all of this is up to you. What do you want to see happen for yourself?"

Ms. D. said, "I care about my [street] family, I care about my [partner], and we drink together. If that's going to kill me, that's going to kill me, but that's my choice." This reminded the addiction psychiatrist and me that our patients, clients, and research participants have their own goals and priorities that we need to honor. We responded that we respected her wishes. We expressed our care and well wishes and left her bedside so she could rest. After our visit, the addiction psychiatrist and I debriefed. He expressed some concerns: Had we done enough? Were we encouraging her use by relenting and not insisting she stop drinking? I understood the concerns and shared his worries but held firm that we needed to honor her wishes and not argue with her about her pathway forward.

A few days after we visited her, we found out that Ms. D. had been released from the hospital. The addiction psychiatrist talked to housing staff, and they agreed he could come by to discuss potential future goals and safer-use strategies with her. When he visited her, he provided Ms. D. with affirmations about the progress she had made to use substances more safely during the study. For example, she had reduced her drinking by a quarter and had stopped injecting heroin. Honoring her desire to continue to use substances socially, he wondered aloud if she could think of a way she could still spend time with her friends and family while intoxicated, but reduce damage to her liver. She seemed intrigued and asked how she might do this. The addiction psychiatrist suggested switching completely to cannabis was one option. She agreed to try that as a safer-use strategy. The addiction psychiatrist worked with housing staff to provide referrals to in-house physicians who could help her obtain a medical marijuana card. Switching to cannabis, Ms. D. continued to reduce her drinking down to about two standard drinks a day. Ms. D. lived for 3 more years in her permanent supportive housing program. When she died, it was at home, on her own terms, and in the arms of "her baby."

Mr. K.

"Mr. K." was a 54-year-old, cisgender, heterosexual, White man who presented for harm reduction treatment (HaRT) in an outpatient addictions clinic. His referral to the HaRT program followed a yearlong, on-and-off engagement in an abstinence-based intensive outpatient treatment program, during which he had a series of escalating verbal altercations with various substance use treatment counselors.

Mr. K.'s substance use assessment indicated current AUD (severe) and intermittent cannabis use. Mr. K. reported engaging in occasional social drinking in his early 20s, with his drinking increasing after his first divorce, in his late 20s and early 30s. He said he would often drink with coworkers after his shifts at the factory where he worked and that his workplace's heavy-drinking culture ended up spilling over into his home life with his second wife and stepdaughter. He indicated this heavy drinking had contributed to his second divorce, loss of his job and home, and resulting estrangement from his parents. A felony arson conviction led to incarceration, and subsequent to his release, he experienced a few years of unsheltered homelessness.

Regarding his prior abstinence-based treatment course, Mr. K. reported he had been frustrated with the substance use treatment counselors and had felt disrespected. He reported feeling particularly angry when substance use treatment counselors would provide a case conceptualization – theorizing about the etiology of his diagnosis, dictating his treatment course, and confronting him about being in denial about his substance use and other aspects of his mental health and identity. After this experience, he reported feeling doubtful about whether substance use treatment could help him. He reported he did not wish to stop drinking or using cannabis but was interested in learning to manage his anger, anxiety, and depression. At the time he started HaRT, he had been working with a harm reduction–oriented housing case manager who had helped him into a Housing First program, which provided permanent, supportive, low-barrier, non-abstinence-based housing. She had encouraged him to engage with HaRT.

Mr. K. provided informed consent to participate in the HaRT protocol outlined in this book. He engaged in weekly, 50-minute outpatient appointments for 2 years, moving to twice a month, 30-minute appointments in the third year. In these sessions, Mr. K. was assessed using the SIP for substance use and substance-related harm, as well as for anxiety (Generalized Anxiety Disorder-7 [GAD-7]) and depression (Patient Health Questionnaire-9 [PHQ-9]). Mr. K. tracked these findings together with the HaRT clinician, developed harm reduction goals and discussed progress made towards them, and committed to safer-use strategies.

Mr. K.'s initial harm reduction goals centered around reducing symptoms of anxiety and depression as well as the negative side effects of alcohol use. Noting a correlation between his experience of substance-related harm and his depressive symptoms, Mr. K. spontaneously expressed an interest in reducing and eventually achieving abstinence from alcohol during the second year of treatment. He also expressed interest in ways of mitigating depressive symptoms, including medications and light therapy. The HaRT clinician encouraged him to use a light box during the darker part of the year and provided a referral to an addiction psychiatrist to prescribe medications to support his harm reduction goals, including managing his alcohol craving (i.e., naltrexone and lamotrigine) and depressive symptoms (i.e., aripiprazole, and trazodone for insomnia). Mid-term harm reduction goals included activities to support his drinking reduction and eventually abstinence-based goals (e.g., journaling, volunteering at a peer-support hotline, attending 12-step groups and church services) and building in positive reinforcement (e.g., eating out, attending baseball games) for treatment gains. As he built this sense of stability, Mr. K.'s goals moved toward achieving greater QoL – attending vocational counseling, getting back into meaningful work, and rebuilding his relationship with his previously estranged children.

Although Mr. K. was not initially interested in changing use, he stopped using alcohol during his second year of treatment, continuing to engage in occasional cannabis use. Although sometimes conflicted about his cannabis use, he has been able to maintain this level of nonproblem use and has a strong relationship with his children and now his grandchildren. He continues to maintain monthly 30-minute harm reduction treatment aftercare meetings to check in about goal setting and achievement as well as overall mental health.

Mr. K. has attributed his improved substance use treatment experience to the low-barrier, flexible, and advocacy-oriented harm reduction approach. His goals drove the eventual assembly of a multidimensional package of services, coordinated by the HaRT clinician and housing case manager. These services supported the client's achievement of his harm reduction goals as they developed over time and included vocational counseling, addiction psychiatry services, and after he attained abstinence, additional substance use counseling that allowed him to work toward regaining his driver's license. Mr. K. appreciated HaRT's flexible, client-driven nature and that harm reduction service providers "reached out of their comfort zone," helping him to set his own goals and advocating for the services he wanted when he was able to engage. Ultimately, the client noted, "It took a village. But harm reduction worked for me. For the first time in my life, I am truly happy."

Postscript

Upon reviewing his case vignette prior to publication, this former client noted that he had developed a cough lately and decided to stop using cannabis. As of this writing, he is 1 month abstinent from cannabis use.

7

Further Reading

Denning, P. & Little, J. (2012). *Practicing harm reduction psychotherapy: An alternative approach to addictions* (2nd ed.). Guilford Press.
The original and groundbreaking harm reduction psychotherapy manual by clinicians for clinicians but steeped in the history and grassroots of harm reduction.

Marlatt, G. A., Witkiewitz, K., & Larimer, M.E. (2011). *Harm reduction: Pragmatic strategies for managing high-risk behaviors* (2nd ed.). Guilford Press.
This edited book considers the evidence base behind harm reduction in the context of various substances and populations.

Marlatt, G. A. (1996). Harm reduction: Come as you are. *Addictive Behaviors, 21,* 779–788.
This classic academic article introduced harm reduction – including its grassroots origins, key definitions, and historical highlights – to the addiction psychology field.

Stout, D. D. (2009). *Coming to harm reduction kicking and screaming: Looking for harm reduction in a 12-step world*. AuthorHouse.
This collection of stories from thought leaders in the field recounts personal and professional experiences with harm reduction and 12-step recovery and points to harm reduction as the future of substance use treatment.

Tartarsky, A. (2002). *Harm reduction psychotherapy: A new treatment for drug and alcohol problems*. Rowman & Littlefield.
One of the original psychotherapeutic contributions to the harm reduction literature, this is a collection of case studies of various clinicians' approaches to harm reduction psychotherapy.

Websites

National Harm Reduction Coalition https://www.harmreduction.org

Harm Reduction International https://hri.global/

Black History Month – The AIDS Network
https://aidsnetwork.ca/blackhistory/

LAC Black Harm Reduction Network
https://www.lac.org/major-project/black-harm-reduction-network

Never Use Alone Inc. https://neverusealone.com/

The People's Harm Reduction Alliance http://phra.org/

Mission of NC Survivors Union http://ncurbansurvivorunion.org/

The Chicago Recovery Alliance http://www.anypositivechange.org

HAMS: Harm Reduction for Alcohol http://hamsnetwork.org/

The Harm Reduction Therapy Center http://www.harmreductiontherapy.org/

HaRRT Center at the University of Washington – Harborview Medical Center https://depts.washington.edu/harrtlab/

HaRT³S http://www.hart3s.com/

Center for Optimal Living https://www.centerforoptimalliving.com/

Drug Policy Alliance http://www.drugpolicy.org/

NEXT Distro https://nextdistro.org/

North American Syringe Exchange Network (NASEN) https://nasen.org/

Self-Help for Clients

Anderson, K. A. (2010). *How to change your drinking: A harm reduction guide to alcohol* (2nd ed.). HAMS Network.

Denning, P., Little, J., & Glickman, A. (Eds.). (2017). *Over the influence: The harm reduction guide to controlling your drug and alcohol* (2nd ed.). Guilford Press.

National Harm Reduction Coalition. (2020). *Getting off right: A safety manual for injection drug users.* Harm Reduction Coalition. https://harmreduction.org/issues/safer-drug-use/injection-safety-manual/

Harm Reduction Resource Center: https://harmreduction.org/our-resources/text-publicationsreports/all-publications/

Harm Reduction History and Broader Aspects

Berridge, V. (1999). Histories of harm reduction: illicit drugs, tobacco, and nicotine. *Substance Use & Misuse, 34*(1), 35–47.

Collins, S. E., Clifasefi, S. L., Logan, D. E., Samples, L., Somers, J., & Marlatt, G. A. (2011). Harm reduction: Current status, historical highlights and basic principles. In G. A. Marlatt, K. Witkiewitz, & M. E. Larimer (Eds.), *Harm reduction: Pragmatic strategies for managing high-risk behaviors* (2nd ed.). Guilford Press. https://www.guilford.com/excerpts/marlatt2.pdf

Grund, J.-P. C., Stern, L. S., Kaplan, C. D., Adriaans, N. F. P., & Drucker, E. (1992). Drug use contexts and HIV-consequences: The effect of drug policy on patterns of everyday drug use in Rotterdam and the Bronx. *British Journal of Addiction, 87*(3), 381–392.

Hart, C. L. (2021). *Drug use for grown-ups: Chasing liberty in the land of fear.* Penguin.

Marlatt, G. A. (1998). Harm reduction around the world: A brief history. In G. A. Marlatt (Ed.), *Harm reduction: Pragmatic strategies for managing high-risk behaviors* (pp. 30–48). Guilford Press.

Maté, G. (2008). *In the realm of hungry ghosts.* North Atlantic Books.

Salavitz, M. (2021). *Undoing drugs: The untold story of harm reduction and the future of addiction.* Hachette.

8

References

Alawadhi, Y. T., Shinagawa, E., Taylor, E. M., Jackson, C., Fragasso, A., Howard, M., Fan, L., Kolpikova, E., Karra, S., Frohe, T., Clifasefi, S. L., Duncan, M. H., & Collins, S. E. (2023). *Safer-use strategies in the context of harm-reduction treatment for people experiencing homelessness and alcohol use disorder* [Manuscript submitted for publication].

Alcoholics Anonymous. (2008). *Alcoholics Anonymous ("The Big Book")* (4th ed.).

American Psychological Association. (2017). *Ethical principles of psychologists and code of conduct* (2002, amended effective June 1, 2010, and January 1, 2017). Retrieved from https://www.apa.org/ethics/code/

Anderson, K. (2010). *How to change your drinking: A harm reduction guide to alcohol.* HAMS Harm Reduction Network.

Angus, C., Latimer, N., Preston, L., Li, J., & Purshouse, R. (2014). What are the implications for policy makers? A systematic review of the cost-effectiveness of screening and brief interventions for alcohol misuse in primary care. *Frontiers in Psychiatry, 5*(114). https://doi.org/10.3389/fpsyt.2014.00114

Becker, H. C. (1998). Kindling in alcohol withdrawal. *Alcohol Health & Research World, 22*(1), 25-33.

Begh, R., Lindson-Hawley, N., & Aveyard, P. (2015). Does reduced smoking if you can't stop make any difference? *BMC Medicine, 13,* 257. https://doi.org/10.1186/s12916-015-0505-2

Bibeau, M., Dionne, F., & Leblanc, J. (2016). Can compassion meditation contribute to the development of psychotherapists' empathy? A review. *Mindfulness, 7*(1), 255-263. https://doi.org/10.1007/s12671-015-0439-y

Bronfenbrenner, U. (1979). *The ecology of human development.* Harvard University Press.

Campinha-Bacote, J. (2019). Cultural competemility: A paradigm shift in the cultural competence versus cultural humility debate – Part I. *Online Journal of Issues in Nursing, 24,* Online publication. https://doi.org/10.3912/OJIN.Vol24No01PPT20

Cepeda, J. A., Eritsyan, K., Vickerman, P., Lyubimova, A., Shegay, M., Odinokova, V., Beletsky, L., Borquez, A., Hickman, M., & Beyrer, C. (2018). Potential impact of implementing and scaling up harm reduction and antiretroviral therapy on HIV prevalence and mortality and overdose deaths among people who inject drugs in two Russian cities: A modelling study. *The Lancet HIV, 5*(10), e578-e587. https://doi.org/10.1016/s2352-3018(18)30168-1

Chang, J. T., Vivar, J. C., Tam, J., Hammad, H. T., Christensen, C. H., van Bemmel, D. M., Das, B., Danilenko, U., & Chang, C. M. (2021). Biomarkers of potential harm among adult cigarette and smokeless tobacco users in the PATH Study Wave 1 (2013-2014): A cross-sectional analysis. *Cancer Epidemiology Biomarkers & Prevention, 30*(7), 1320-1327. https://doi.org/10.1158/1055-9965.Epi-20-1544

Chimbar, L., & Moleta, Y. (2018). Naloxone effectiveness: A systematic review. *Journal of Addictions Nursing, 29*(3), 167-171. https://doi.org/10.1097/jan.0000000000000230

Clifasefi, S. L., Collins, S. E., Torres, N. I., Grazioli, V. S., & Mackelprang, J. L. (2016). Housing First, but what comes second? A qualitative study of resident, staff and management perspectives on single-site Housing First program enhancement. *Journal of Community Psychology, 44*(7), 845-855. https://doi.org/10.1002/jcop.21812

Clifasefi, S. L., Lonczak, H. S., & Collins, S. E. (2017). Seattle's Law Enforcement Assisted Diversion (LEAD) program: Within-subjects changes on housing, employment, and income/benefits outcomes and associations with recidivism. *Crime & Delinquency, 63*(4), 429–445. https://doi.org/10.1177/0011128716687550

Clifasefi, S. L., Malone, D., & Collins, S. E. (2013). Associations between criminal history, housing first exposure and jail outcomes among chronically homeless individuals with alcohol problems. *International Journal of Drug Policy, 24,* 291–296. https://doi.org/10.1016/j.drugpo.2012.10.002

Collins, S. E. (2016). Associations between socioeconomic factors and alcohol outcomes. *Alcohol Research: Current Reviews, 38*(1), 83–94. https://pubmed.ncbi.nlm.nih.gov/27159815

Collins, S. E., Black Bear, L., Buffalomeat, S., Fields, R., Lumsden, J. S., Mayberry, N., Rosario, J., Stanton, J., & Williams, G. (2018, June 8). *Where harm reduction meets Housing First: Exploring alcohol use among residents in a project-based Housing First program* [Paper presentation]. Grand Rounds in the Department of Psychiatry and Behavioral Sciences at the University of Washington Medical School, Seattle, WA, USA. https://depts.washington.edu/harrtlab/577/psychiatry-behavioral-sciences-grand-rounds-6-8-2018/

Collins, S. E., Carey, K. B., & Sliwinski, M. J. (2002). Mailed personalized normative feedback as a brief intervention for at-risk college drinkers. *Journal of Studies on Alcohol, 63,* 559–567. https://doi.org/10.15288/jsa.2002.63.559

Collins, S. E., Clifasefi, S. L., Andrasik, M. P., Dana, E. A., Stahl, N. E., Kirouac, M., Welbaum, C., King, M., & Malone, D. K. (2012). Exploring transitions within a project-based Housing First setting: Qualitative evaluation and practice implications. *Journal of Health Care for the Poor and Underserved, 23,* 1678–1697. https://doi.org/10.1353/hpu.2012.0187

Collins, S. E., Clifasefi, S. L., Dana, E. A., Andrasik, M. P., Stahl, N. E., Kirouac, M., Welbaum, C., King, M., & Malone, D. K. (2012). Where harm reduction meets Housing First: Exploring alcohol's role in a project-based Housing First setting. *International Journal of Drug Policy, 23,* 111–119. https://doi.org/10.1016/j.drugpo.2011.07.010

Collins, S. E., Clifasefi, S. L., Logan, D. E., Samples, L., Somers, J., & Marlatt, G. A. (2011). Harm reduction: Current status, historical highlights and basic principles. In G. A. Marlatt, K. Witkiewitz, & M. E. Larimer (Eds.), *Harm reduction: Pragmatic strategies for managing high-risk behaviors* (2nd ed.). Guilford Press. https://www.guilford.com/excerpts/marlatt2.pdf

Collins, S. E., Clifasefi, S. L., Nelson, L. A., Stanton, J., Goldstein, S. C., Taylor, E. M., Hoffmann, G., King, V. L., Hatsukami, A. S., Cunningham, Z. L., Taylor, E., Mayberry, N., Malone, D. K., & Jackson, T. R. (2019). Randomized controlled trial of Harm Reduction Treatment for Alcohol (HaRT-A) for people experiencing homelessness and alcohol use disorder. *International Journal of Drug Policy, 67,* 24–33.

Collins, S. E., Clifasefi, S. L., Stanton, J., The LEAP Advisory Board, Straits, K. J. E., Gil-Kashiwabara, E., Rodriguez Espinosa, P., Nicasio, A. V., Andrasik, M. P., Hawes, S. M., Miller, K. A., Nelson, L. A., Orfaly, V. E., Duran, B. M., & Wallerstein, N. (2018). Community-based participatory research (CBPR): Towards equitable involvement of community in psychology research. *American Psychologist, 73,* 884–898. https://doi.org/10.1037/amp0000167

Collins, S. E., Clifasefi, S. L., Williams, G. W., Black Bear, L., & The LEAP Community Advisory Board. (2022). Community-based harm reduction approaches for alcohol use disorder. In J. A. Tucker & K. Witkiewitz (Eds.), *Dynamic pathways to recovery from alcohol use disorder* (pp. 218–238). Cambridge University Press.

Collins, S. E., Duncan, M. H., Saxon, A. J., Merrill, J. O., & Ries, R. K. (2016). Substance use disorders: Alcohol, stimulants and opioids. In A. Ratzliff, J. Unützer, W. Katon, & K. A. Stephens (Eds.), *Integrated care: Creating effective mental and primary health care teams* (pp. 124–152). Wiley. https://doi.org/10.1002/9781119276579.ch6

Collins, S. E., Duncan, M. H., Saxon, A. J., Taylor, E. M., Mayberry, N., Merrill, J. O., Hoffmann, G. E., Clifasefi, S. L., & Ries, R. K. (2021). Combining behavioral harm-reduction treatment and extended-release naltrexone for people experiencing homelessness and alcohol use disorder in the USA: A randomised clinical trial. *Lancet Psychiatry, 8*(4), 287-300. https://doi.org/10.1016/s2215-0366(20)30489-2

Collins, S. E., Duncan, M. H., Smart, B. F., Saxon, A. J., Malone, D., Jackson, T., & Ries, R. (2015). Extended-release naltrexone and harm reduction counseling for chronically homeless people with alcohol dependence. *Substance Abuse, 36,* 21-33. https://doi.org/10.1080/08897077.2014.904838

Collins, S. E., Eck, S., Torchalla, I., Schröter, M., & Batra, A. (2013). Understanding treatment-seeking smokers' motivation to change: Content analysis of the decisional balance worksheet. *Addictive Behaviors, 38*(1), 1472-1480. https://doi.org/https://doi.org/10.1016/j.addbeh.2012.08.008

Collins, S. E., Goldstein, S. C., King, V. L., Orfaly, V. E., Gu, J., Clark, A., Vess, A., Lee, G., Taylor, E. M., Fentress, T., Braid, A. K., & Clifasefi, S. L. (2021). Characterizing components of and attendance at resident-driven Housing First programming in the context of community-based participatory research. *Journal of Community Psychology, 49*(5), 1376-1392. https://doi.org/https://doi.org/10.1002/jcop.22491

Collins, S. E., Goldstein, S. C., Suprasert, B., Doerr, S. A. M., Gliane, J., Song, C., Orfaly, V. E., Moodliar, R., Taylor, E. M., & Hoffmann, G. (2021). Jail and emergency department utilization in the context of harm reduction treatment for people experiencing homelessness and alcohol use disorder. *Journal of Urban Health, 98,* 83-90. https://doi.org/10.1007/s11524-020-00452-8

Collins, S. E., Grazioli, V., Torres, N., Taylor, E., Jones, C., Hoffman, G., Haelsig, L., Zhu, M., Hatsukami, D., Koker, M., Herndon, P., Greenleaf, S., & Dean, P. (2015). Qualitatively and quantitatively defining harm-reduction goals among chronically homeless individuals with alcohol dependence. *Addictive Behaviors, 45,* 184-190.

Collins, S. E., Jones, C. B., Hoffmann, G., Nelson, L. A., Hawes, S. M., Grazioli, V. S., Mackelprang, J. L., Holttum, J., Kaese, G., Lenert, J., Herndon, P., & Clifasefi, S. L. (2016). In their own words: Content analysis of pathways to recovery among individuals with the lived experience of homelessness and alcohol use disorders. *International Journal on Drug Policy, 27,* 89-96. https://doi.org/10.1016/j.drugpo.2015.08.003

Collins, S. E., Kirouac, M., Taylor, E., Spelman, P. J., Grazioli, V., Hoffman, G., Haelsig, L., Holttum, J., Kanagawa, A., Nehru, M., & Hicks, J. (2014). Advantages and disadvantages of college drinking in students' own words: Content analysis of the decisional balance worksheet. *Psychology of Addictive Behaviors, 28*(3), 727-733. https://doi.org/10.1037/a0036354

Collins, S. E., Lonczak, H. S., & Clifasefi, S. L. (2017). Seattle's Law Enforcement Assisted Diversion (LEAD): Program effects on recidivism outcomes. *Evaluation and Program Planning, 64,* 49-56. https://doi.org/10.1016/j.evalprogplan.2017.05.008

Collins, S. E., Malone, D. K., & Larimer, M. E. (2012). Motivation to change and treatment attendance as predictors of alcohol-use outcomes among project-based housing first residents. *Addictive Behaviors, 37,* 931-939. https://doi.org/10.1016/j.addbeh.2012.03.029

Collins, S. E., Nelson, L. A., Stanton, J., Mayberry, N., Ubay, T., Taylor, E. M., Hoffmann, G., Goldstein, S. C., Saxon, A. J., Malone, D. M., Clifasefi, S. L., Okuyemi, K., & the HaRT-S Community Advisory Board. (2019). Harm reduction treatment for smoking (HaRT-S): Findings from a single-arm pilot study with smokers experiencing chronic homelessness. *Substance Abuse, 40,* 229-239. https://doi.org/10.1080/08897077.2019.1572049

Collins, S. E., Orfaly, V. E., Wu, T., Chang, S., Hardy, R. V., Nash, A., Jones, M. B., Mares, L., Taylor, E. M., Nelson, L. A., & Clifasefi, S. L. (2018). Content analysis of homeless smokers' perspectives on established and alternative smoking interventions. *International Journal of Drug Policy, 51,* 10-17. https://doi.org/10.1016/j.drugpo.2017.09.007

Collins, S. E., Saxon, A. J., Duncan, M. H., Smart, B. F., Merrill, J. O., Malone, D. K., Jackson, T. R., Clifasefi, S. L., Joesch, J., & Ries, R. K. (2014). Harm reduction with pharmacotherapy for homeless people with alcohol dependence: Protocol for a randomized controlled trial. *Contemporary Clinical Trials, 38*, 221–234. https://doi.org/10.1016/j.cct.2014.05.008

Collins, S. E., Taylor, E., Jones, C., Haelsig, L., Grazioli, V. S., Mackelprang, J. L., Holttum, J., Koker, M., Hatsukami, A., & Baker, M. (2018). Content analysis of advantages and disadvantages of drinking among individuals with the lived experience of homelessness and alcohol use disorders. *Substance Use & Misuse, 53*(1), 16–25. https://doi.org/10.1080/10826084.2017.1322406

Cooper, R. L., Ramesh, A., Juarez, P. D., Edgerton, R., Paul, M., Tabatabai, M., Brown, K. Y., & Matthews-Juarez, P. (2020). Systematic review of opioid use disorder treatment training for medical students and residents. *Journal of Health Care for the Poor and Underserved, 31*(5), 26–42. https://doi.org/10.1353/hpu.2020.0136

Crabtree, A., Latham, N., Morgan, R., Pauly, B., Bungay, V., & Buxton, J. A. (2018). Perceived harms and harm reduction strategies among people who drink non-beverage alcohol: Community-based qualitative research in Vancouver, Canada. *International Journal of Drug Policy, 59*, 85–93. https://doi.org/10.1016/j.drugpo.2018.06.020

Degenhardt, L., Mathers, B., Vickerman, P., Rhodes, T., Latkin, C., & Hichkman, M. (2010). Prevention of HIV infection for people who inject drugs: Why individual, structural, and combination approaches are needed. *Lancet, 376*, 285–301. https://doi.org/10.1016/S01406736(10)60742-8

Denning, P. (2010). Harm reduction therapy with families and friends of people with drug problems. *Journal of Clinical Psychology, 66*, 164–174. https://doi.org/10.1002/jclp.20671

Denning, P., & Little, J. (2012). *Practicing harm reduction psychotherapy: An alternative approach to addictions* (2nd ed.). Guilford Press.

Denning, P., & Little, J. (Eds.). (2017). *Over the influence: The harm reduction guide for managing drugs and alcohol*. Guilford Press.

Dickerson, D. L., Brown, R. A., Johnson, C. L., Schweigman, K., & D'Amico, E. J. (2016). Integrating motivational interviewing and traditional practices to address alcohol and drug use among urban American Indian/Alaska Native youth. *Journal of Substance Abuse Treatment, 65*, 26–35. https://doi.org/10.1016/j.jsat.2015.06.023

Dimeff, L. A., Baer, J. S., Kivlahan, D. R., & Marlatt, G. A. (1999). *Brief alcohol screening and intervention for college students (BASICS): A harm reduction approach*. Guilford Press.

Duran, B. (1996). Indigenous versus colonial discourse: Alcohol and American Indian identity. In E. Bird (Ed.), *Dressing in feathers: The construction of the Indian in American popular culture* (pp. 111–128). Westview Press.

Earnshaw, V. A. (2020). Stigma and substance use disorders: A clinical, research, and advocacy agenda. *American Psychologist, 75*(9), 1300–1311. https://doi.org/10.1037/amp0000744

Earp, B. D., Lewis, J., & Hart, C. L. (2021). Racial justice requires ending the war on drugs. *American Journal of Bioethics, 21*(4), 4–19. https://doi.org/10.1080/15265161.2020.1861364

Fachini, A., Aliane, P. P., Martinez, E. Z., & Furtado, E. F. (2012). Efficacy of brief alcohol screening intervention for college students (BASICS): A meta-analysis of randomized controlled trials. *Substance Abuse Treatment, Prevention, and Policy, 7*(1), 40. https://doi.org/10.1186/1747-597X-7-40

Fentress, T., Wald, S., Brah, A., Leemon, G., Reyes, R., Alkhamees, F., Kramer, M., Taylor, E. M., Wildwood, M., Frohe, T., Duncan, M. H., Clifasefi, S. L., & Collins, S. E. (2021). Dual study defining patient-driven harm reduction goal-setting among people experiencing homelessness and alcohol use disorder. *Experimental and Clinical Psychopharmacology, 29*, 261–271.

Goldstein, S. C., Weiss, N. H., Yang, M., Feldstein-Ewing, S., & Collins, S. E. (2023). *Testing race, ethnicity, and sex assigned at birth as moderators of harm reduction pharmacobehavioral treatment outcomes for alcohol use disorder among people experiencing homelessness* [Manuscript submitted for publication].

Grazioli, V. S., Collins, S. E., Daeppen, J.-B., & Larimer, M. E. (2014). Perceptions of alcoholics anonymous among chronically homeless individuals with alcohol-use disorders. *International Journal of Drug Policy, 26*, 468–474. https://doi.org/10.1016/j.drugpo.2014.10.009

Grazioli, V. S., Hicks, J., Kaese, G., Lenert, J., & Collins, S. E. (2015). Safer-drinking strategies used by chronically homeless individuals with alcohol dependence. *Journal of Substance Abuse Treatment, 54*, 63–68. https://doi.org/10.1016/j.jsat.2015.01.010

Grouzet, F. M. E., Kasser, T., Ahuvia, A., Dols, J. M. F., Kim, Y., Lau, S., Ryan, R. M., Saunders, S., Schmuck, P., & Sheldon, K. M. (2005). The structure of goal contents across 15 cultures. *Journal of Personality and Social Psychology, 89*, 800–816. https://doi.org/http://dx.doi.org/10.1037/0022-3514.89.5.800

Guerra-Doce, E. (2015). Psychoactive substances in prehistoric times: Examining the archaeological evidence. *Time and Mind, 8*(1), 91–112. https://doi.org/10.1080/1751696X.2014.993244

Hagman, B. T., Falk, D., Litten, R., & Koob, G. F. (2022). Defining recovery from alcohol use disorder: Development of an NIAAA research definition. *American Journal of Psychiatry*. Advance online publication. https://doi.org/10.1176/appi.ajp.21090963

Hart, C. L. (2021). *Drug use for grown-ups: Chasing liberty in the land of fear*. Penguin.

Haug, N. A., Morimoto, E. E., & Lembke, A. (2020). Online mutual-help intervention for reducing heavy alcohol use. *Journal of Addictive Diseases, 38*(3), 241–249. https://doi.org/10.1080/10550887.2020.1747331

Hawk, M., Coulter, R. W. S., Egan, J. E., Fisk, S., Reuel Friedman, M., Tula, M., & Kinsky, S. (2017). Harm reduction principles for healthcare settings. *Harm reduction journal, 14*(1), 70-70. https://doi.org/10.1186/s12954-017-0196-4

Heather, N. (2006). Controlled drinking, harm reduction and their roles in the response to alcohol-related problems. *Addiction Research and Theory, 14*, 7–18. https://doi.org/10.1080/16066350500489170

Heilig, M., MacKillop, J., Martinez, D., Rehm, J., Leggio, L., & Vanderschuren, L. J. M. J. (2021). Addiction as a brain disease revised: Why it still matters, and the need for consilience. *Neuropsychopharmacology, 46*, 1715–1723. https://doi.org/10.1038/s41386-020-00950-y

Hwang, S. W., Tolomiczenko, G., Kouyoumdjian, F. G., & Garner, R. E. (2006). Interventions to improve the health of the homeless. *American Journal of Preventative Medicine, 29*, 311–319.

Kahn, C. B., Reinschmidt, K., Teufel-Shone, N. I., Oré, C. E., Henson, M., & Attakai, A. (2016). American Indian Elders' resilience: Sources of strength for building a healthy future for youth. *American Indian and Alaska Native Mental Health Research (Online), 23*(3), 117–133. https://doi.org/10.5820/aian.2303.2016.117

Kelly, J. F., & Westerhoff, C. M. (2010). Does it matter how we refer to individuals with substance-related conditions? A randomized study of two commonly used terms. *International Journal of Drug Policy, 21*, 202–207. https://doi.org/https://doi.org/10.1016/j.drugpo.2009.10.010

Klimecki, O. M., Leiberg, S., Ricard, M., & Singer, T. (2013). Differential pattern of functional brain plasticity after compassion and empathy training. *Social Cognitive and Affective Neuroscience, 9*(6), 873–879. https://doi.org/10.1093/scan/nst060

Kulesza, M., Larimer, M. E., & Rao, D. (2013). Substance use related stigma: What we know and the way forward. *Journal of Addictive Behaviors, Therapy & Rehabilitation, 2*(2), 782. https://doi.org/10.4172/2324-9005.1000106

Larimer, M. E., & Cronce, J. M. (2007). Identification, prevention, and treatment revisited: Individual-focused college drinking prevention strategies 1999–2006.

Addictive Behavior, 32, 2439–2468. https://doi.org/2410.1016/j.addbeh.2007.2405.2006

Larimer, M., Malone, D., Garner, M., Atkins, D., Burlingham, B., Lonczak, H., Tanzer, K., Ginzler, J., Clifasefi, S. L., Hobson, W. G., & Marlatt, G. A. (2009). Health care and public service use and costs before and after provision of housing for chronically homeless persons with severe alcohol problems. *JAMA, 301*, 1349–1357. https://doi.org/10.1001/jama.2009.414

Layton, J. (2005). *How fear works.* Howstuffworks. https://science.howstuffworks.com/life/inside-the-mind/emotions/fear.htm

Ledesma, R. (2007). The urban Los Angeles American Indian experience: Perspectives from the field. *Journal of Ethnic & Cultural Diversity in Social Work, 16*(1-2), 27–60. https://doi.org/10.1300/J051v16n01_02

Lee, P. N. (2013). The effect on health of switching from cigarettes to snus – A review. *Regulatory Toxicology and Pharmacology, 66*(1), 1–5. https://doi.org/10.1016/j.yrtph.2013.02.010

Lee, H. S., & Petersen, S. R. (2009). Demarginalizing the marginalized in substance abuse treatment: Stories of homeless, active substance users in an urban harm reduction based drop-in center. *Addiction Research & Theory, 17*(6), 622–636. https://doi.org/10.3109/16066350802168613

Legha, R., Raleigh-Cohn, A., Fickenscher, A., & Novins, D. K. (2014). Challenges to providing quality substance abuse treatment services for American Indian and Alaska Native communities: Perspectives of staff from 18 treatment centers. *BMC Psychiatry,* 14. https://www.biomedcentral.com/1471-1244X/1414/1181 https://doi.org/10.1186/1471-244X-14-181

Leong, F. T., & Park, Y. S. (2016). Introduction. In Council of National Psychological Associations for the Advancement of Ethnic Minority Interests. (Ed.), *Testing and assessment with persons & communities of color.* American Psychological Association.

Leshner, A. I. (1997). Addiction is a brain disease and it matters. *Science, 278*, 45–47. https://doi.org/10.1126/science.1278.5335.1145

Lovibond, S. H., & Caddy, G. (1970). Discriminative aversive control in the moderation of alcoholics' drinking behavior. *Behavior Therapy, 24*, 461–504.

Ma, J., Bao, Y.-P., Wang, R.-J., Su, M.-F., Liu, M.-X., Li, J.-Q., Degenhardt, L., Farrell, M., Blow, F. C., & Ilgen, M. (2019). Effects of medication-assisted treatment on mortality among opioids users: a systematic review and meta-analysis. *Molecular Psychiatry, 24*(12), 1868–1883. https://doi.org/10.1038/s41380-018-0094-5

Mackelprang, J. L., Collins, S. E., & Clifasefi, S. L. (2014). Housing First is associated with reduced use of emergency medical services. *Prehospital Emergency Care,* 18. https://doi.org/10.3109/10903127.2014.916020

Maglione, M. A., Raaen, L., Chen, C., Azhar, G., Shahidinia, N., Shen, M., Maksabedian, E., Shanman, R. M., Newberry, S., & Hempel, S. (2018). Effects of medication assisted treatment (MAT) for opioid use disorder on functional outcomes: A systematic review. *Journal of Substance Abuse Treatment, 89*, 28–51. https://doi.org/10.7249/RR2108

Malone, D. K., Collins, S. E., & Clifasefi, S. L. (2015). Single-site Housing First for chronically homeless people. *Housing, Care and Support, 18*, 62–66. https://doi.org/10.1108/HCS-05-2015-0007

Marlatt, G. A. (1996). Harm reduction: Come as you are. *Addictive Behaviors, 21*, 779–788. https://doi.org/10.1016/0306-4603(96)00042-1

Marlatt, G. A. (1998a). Basic principles and strategies of harm reduction. In G. A. Marlatt (Ed.), *Harm reduction: Pragmatic strategies for managing high-risk behaviors* (pp. 49–66). Guilford Press.

Marlatt, G. A. (1998b). Highlights of harm reduction: A personal report from the First National Harm Reduction Conference in the US. In G. A. Marlatt (Ed.), *Harm reduction: Pragmatic strategies for managing high-risk behaviors.* Guilford Press.

Marlatt, G. A., & Gordon, J. R. (1985). *Relapse prevention: Maintenance strategies in the treatment of addictive behaviors.* Guilford Press.

Marlatt, G. A., Larimer, M. E., Baer, J. S., & Quigley, L. A. (1993). Harm reduction for alcohol problems: Moving beyond the controlled drinking controversy. *Behavior Therapy, 24,* 461–504. https://doi.org/10.1016/S0005-7894(05)80314-4

Marlatt, G. A., & Witkiewitz, K. (2002). Harm reduction approaches to alcohol use: Health promotion, prevention, and treatment. *Addictive Behaviors, 27*(6), 867–886. https://doi.org/10.1016/s0306-4603(02)00294-0

Marlatt, G. A., & Witkiewitz, K. (2010). Update on harm-reduction policy and intervention research. *Annual Review of Clinical Psychology, 6,* 591–606. https://doi.org/10.1146/annurev.clinpsy.121208.131438

McCambridge, J., & Saitz, R. (2017). Rethinking brief interventions for alcohol in general practice. *BMJ, 356.* https://doi.org/10.1136/bmj.j116

McLellan, A. T., Koob, G. F., & Volkow, N. D. (2022). Preaddiction: A missing concept for treating substance use disorders. *JAMA Psychiatry, 79*(8), 749–751. https://doi.org/10.1001/jamapsychiatry.2022.1652

McLellan, A. T., Kushner, H., Metzger, D., & Peters, R. (1992). The fifth edition of the Addiction Severity Index. *Journal of Substance Abuse Treatment, 9,* 199–213. https://doi.org/10.1016/0740-5472(92)90062-S

Miller, W. R. (1996). Motivational interviewing: Research, practice, and puzzles. *Addictive Behaviors, 21,* 835–842. https://doi.org/10.1016/0306-4603(96)00044-5

Miller, W. R., Moyers, T., Arciniega, L., Ernst, D. B., & Forcehimes, A. (2005). Training, supervision and quality monitoring of the COMBINE Study behavioral interventions. *Journal of Studies on Alcohol, s15,* 188–195. https://doi.org/10.15288/jsas.2005.s15.188

Miller, W. R., & Rollnick, S. (2009). Ten things that motivational interviewing is not. *Behavioural and Cognitive Psychotherapy, 37*(2), 129–140. https://doi.org/10.1017/S1352465809005128

Miller, W. R., & Rollnick, S. (2013). *Motivational interviewing: Helping people change* (3rd ed.). Guilford Press.

Miller, W. R., Tonigan, J., & Longabaugh, R. (1995). *The Drinker Inventory of Consequences (DrInC): An instrument for assessing adverse consequences of alcohol abuse. Test manual* (NIH Publication No. 95-3911). US Department of Health and Human Services, Public Health Service, National Institutes of Health, National Institute on Alcohol Abuse and Alcoholism. https://pubs.niaaa.nih.gov/publications/projectmatch/match04.pdf

Mostofi, N., & Collins, S. E. (in press). Impact of harm reduction treatment with or without pharmacotherapy on concurrent substance use among people experiencing homelessness and alcohol use disorder. *Journal of Addiction Medicine.*

National Academies of Sciences Engineering and Medicine. (2018). Harm reduction. In *Public health consequences of e-cigarettes* (pp. 18.11–18.34). National Academies Press. https://doi.org/10.17226/24952

National Harm Reduction Coalition. (2020). *Getting off right: A safety manual for injection drug users.* https://harmreduction.org/wp-content/uploads/2020/08/Resource-SaferDruguse-GettingOffRightASafetyManualforInjectionDrugUsers.pdf

National Institute on Drug Abuse. (2008). *Drugs, brains and behavior: The science of addiction* (NIH Publication No. 07-5605). National Institutes of Health.

Nelson, L. A., Collins, S. E., Birch, J., Burns, R., McPhail, G., Onih, J., Cupp, C., Ubay, T., King, V., Taylor, E., Masciel, K., Slaney, T., Bunch, J., King, R., Piper, B. K. S., & Squetimkin-Anquoe, A. (2023). Content analysis of preferred recovery pathways among urban American Indians and Alaska Natives experiencing alcohol use disorders. *Journal of Cross Cultural Psychology, 54*(1), 142–160. https://doi.org/10.1177/00220221221132778

Nelson, L. A., Squetimkin-Anquoe, A., Ubay, T., King, V., Taylor, E. M., Masciel, K., Black Bear, L., Buffalomeat, S., Duffing-Romero, X., Garza, C. M., Clifasefi, S. L., & Collins, S. E. (2022). Content analysis informing the development of adapted harm reduction Talking Circles (HaRTC) with urban American Indians and Alaska Natives experiencing alcohol use disorder. *International Journal of Indigenous Health, 17*(2), 33–50. https://doi.org/https://doi.org/10.32799/ijih.v17i2.36677

Novins, D. K., Aarons, G. A., Conti, S. G., Dahlke, D., Daw, R., Fickenscher, A., Fleming, C., Love, C., Masis, K., Spicer, P., & The Centers for American Indian and Alaska Native Health's Substance Abuse Treatment Advisory Board. (2011). Use of the evidence base in substance abuse treatment programs for American Indians and Alaska Natives: Pursuing quality in the crucible of practice and policy. *Implementation Science, 6*. https://doi.org/10.1186/1748-5908-6-63

Novins, D. K., Croy, C. D., Moore, L. A., & Rieckmann, T. (2016). Use of evidence-based treatments in substance abuse treatment programs serving American Indian and Alaska Native communities. *Drug Alcohol Dependence, 161*, 214–221. https://doi.org/10.1016/j.drugalcdep.2016.02.007

Nutt, D. J., Phillips, L. D., Balfour, D., Curran, H. V., Dockrell, M., Foulds, J., Fagerstrom, K., Letlape, K., Milton, A., Polosa, R., Ramsey, J., & Sweanor, D. (2014). Estimating the harms of nicotine-containing products using the MCDA approach. *European Addiction Research, 20*(5), 218–225. https://www.karger.com/DOI/10.1159/000360220 https://doi.org/10.1159/000360220

O'Donnell, A., Anderson, P., Newbury-Birch, D., Schulte, B., Schmidt, C., Reimer, J., & Kaner, E. (2013). The impact of brief alcohol interventions in primary healthcare: A systematic review of reviews. *Alcohol and Alcoholism, 49*(1), 66–78. https://doi.org/10.1093/alcalc/agt170

Orwin, R. G., Garrison-Mogren, R., Jacobs, M. L., & Sonnefeld, L. J. (1999). Retention of homeless clients in substance abuse treatment: Findings from the National Institute on Alcohol Abuse and Alcoholism Cooperative Agreement Program. *Journal of Substance Abuse Treatment, 17*, 45–66. https://doi.org/10.1016/S0740-5472(98)00046-4

Pauly, B., Vallance, K., Wettlaufer, A., Chow, C., Brown, R., Evans, J., Gray, E., Krysowaty, B., Ivsins, A., & Schiff, R. (2018). Community managed alcohol programs in Canada: Overview of key dimensions and implementation. *Drug and Alcohol Review, 37*, S132–S139. https://doi.org/10.1111/dar.12681

Pearson, M. R. (2013). Use of alcohol protective behavioral strategies among college students: A critical review. *Clinical Psychology Review, 33*, https://doi.org/10.1016/j.cpr.2013.08.006

Pettinati, H. M., Weiss, R. D., Miller, W. R., Donovan, D. M., Ernst, D. B., & Rounsaville, B. J. (2004). *Medical management treatment manual: A clinical research guide for medically trained clinicians providing pharmacotherapy as part of a treatment for alcohol dependence* (Vol. 2; COMBINE Monograph Series; DHHS Publication No. 04-5289). National Institute on Alcohol Abuse and Alcoholism.

Pisinger, C., & Godtfredsen, N. S. (2007). Is there a health benefit of reduced tobacco consumption? A systematic review. *Nicotine and Tobacco Research, 9*, 631–646. https://doi.org/10.1080/14622200701365327

Ray, L. A., Bujarski, S., Grodin, E., Hartwell, E., Green, R., Venegas, A., Lim, A. C., Gillis, A., & Miotto, K. (2019). State-of-the-art behavioral and pharmacological treatments for alcohol use disorder. *American Journal of Drug and Alcohol Abuse, 45*, 124–140. https://doi.org/10.1080/00952990.2018.1528265

Reinschmidt, K. M., Attakai, A., Kahn, C. B., Whitewater, S., & Teufel-Shone, N. (2016). Shaping a stories of resilience model from urban American Indian elders' narratives of historical trauma and resilience. *American Indian and Alaska Native Mental Health Research, 23*(4), 63–85. https://doi.org/10.5820/aian.2304.2016.63

Rezk-Hanna, M., Warda, U. S., Stokes, A. C., Fetterman, J., Li, J., Macey, P. M., Darawad, M., Song, Y., Ben Taleb, Z., Brecht, M.-L., & Benowitz, N. L. (2022). Associations of smokeless tobacco use with cardiovascular disease risk: Insights from the Population Assessment of Tobacco and Health Study. *Nicotine & Tobacco Research, 24*(7), 1063–1070. https://doi.org/10.1093/ntr/ntab258

Rogers, C. R. (1957). The necessary and sufficient conditions of therapeutic personality change. *Journal of Consulting Psychology, 21*, 95–103. https://doi.org/10.1037/h0045357

Rosenheck, R. A., Morrissey, J., Lam, J., Calloway, M., Johnsen, M., Goldman, H., Randolph, F., Blasinsky, M., Fontana, A., Calsyn, R., & Teague, G. (1998). Service system integration, access to services, and housing outcomes in a program for homeless persons with severe mental illness. *American Journal of Public Health, 88,* 1610-1615. https://doi.org/10.2105/AJPH.88.11.1610

Smith, J. E., Meyers, R. J., & Delaney, H. D. (1998). The Community Reinforcement Approach with homeless alcohol-dependent individuals. *Journal of Consulting and Clinical Psychology, 66,* 541-548. https://doi.org/10.1037//0022-006X.66.3.541

Sobell, L. C., Ellingstad, T. P., & Sobell, M. B. (2000). Natural recovery from alcohol and drug problems: Methodological review of the research with suggestions for future directions. *Addiction, 95*(5), 749-764. https://doi.org/10.1046/j.1360-0443.2000.95574911.x

Sobell, L. C., & Sobell, M. B. (1992). Timeline followback: A technique for assessing self-reported ethanol consumption. In J. Allen & R. Z. Litten (Eds.), *Measuring alcohol consumption: Psychosocial and biological methods* (pp. 41-72). Humana Press.

Sobell, M. B., & Sobell, L. C. (1973a). Alcoholics treated by individualized behavior therapy: One year treatment outcome. *Behaviour Research and Therapy, 11,* 599-618. https://doi.org/10.1016/0005-7967(73)90118-6

Sobell, M. B., & Sobell, L. C. (1973b). Individualized behavior therapy for alcoholics. *Behavior Therapy, 4,* 49-72. https://doi.org/10.1016/S0005-7894(73)80074-7

Sobell, M. B., & Sobell, L. C. (1976). Second year treatment outcome of alcoholics treated by individualized behavior therapy: Results. *Behavioral Research and Therapy, 14,* 195-215. https://doi.org/10.1016/0005-7967(76)90013-9

Sobell, M. B., & Sobell, L. C. (1995). Controlled drinking after 25 years: How important was the great debate? *Addiction, 90,* 1149-1153. https://doi.org/10.1111/j.1360-0443.1995.tb01077.x

Sobell, M. B., & Sobell, L. C. (2005). Guided self-change model of treatment for substance use disorders. *Journal of Cognitive Psychotherapy, 19,* 199-210. https://doi.org/10.1891/jcop.2005.19.3.199

Stahl, N., Collins, S. E., Clifasefi, S. L., & Hagopian, A. (2016). When Housing First lasts: Exploring the lived experience of single-site Housing First residents. *Journal of Community Psychology, 44,* 848-498. https://doi.org/10.1002/jcop.21783

Stergiopoulos, V., Gozdzik, A., Misir, V., Skosireva, A., Connelly, J., Sarang, A., Whisler, A., Hwang, S. W., O'Campo, P., & McKenzic, K. (2015). Effectiveness of Housing First with intensive case managment in an ethnically diverse sample of homeless adults with mental illness: A randomized controlled trial. *PLoS One, 10,* e0130281.

Stockwell, T., Pauly, B., Chow, C., Erickson, R. A., Krysowaty, B., Roemer, A., Vallance, K., Wettlaufer, A., & Zhao, J. (2018). Does managing the consumption of people with severe alcohol dependence reduce harm? A comparison of participants in six Canadian managed alcohol programs with locally recruited controls. *Drug and Alcohol Review, 37,* S159-S166. https://doi.org/10.1111/dar.12618

Substance Abuse and Mental Health Services Administration. (1999). *Enhancing motivation for change in substance abuse treatment* (DHHS Publication No. SMA 00-3460).

Substance Abuse and Mental Health Services Administration (SAMHSA). (2022). *Key substance use and mental health indicators in the United States: Results from the 2021 National Survey on Drug Use and Health* (HHS Publication No. PEP22-07-01-005, NSDUH Series H-57). https://www.samhsa.gov/data/report/2021-nsduh-annual-national-report

Sue, D. W. (2003). Cultural competence in the treatment of ethnic minority populations. In D. W. Sue (Ed.), *Psychological treatment of ethnic minority populations.* Association of Black Psychologists.

Szalavitz, M. (2021). *Undoing drugs: The untold story of harm reduction and the future of addiction.* Go Hachette Books.

Tartarsky, A. (2002). *Harm reduction psychotherapy: A new treatment for drug and alcohol problems.* Rowman & Littlefield.

Tervalon, M., & Murray-Garcia, J. (1998). Cultural humility vs. cultural competence: A critical distinction in defining physician training outcomes in medical education. *Journal of Health Care for the Poor and Underserved, 9*, 117-125.

Timko, C., Schultz, N. R., Cucciare, M. A., Vittorio, L., & Garrison-Diehn, C. (2016). Retention in medication-assisted treatment for opiate dependence: A systematic review. *Journal of Addictive Diseases, 35*(1), 22-35. https://doi.org/10.1080/10550887.2016.1100960

Tkacz, J., Severt, J., Cacciola, J., & Ruetsch, C. (2012). Compliance with buprenorphine medication-assisted treatment and relapse to opioid use. *American Journal on Addictions, 21*(1), 55-62. https://doi.org/https://doi.org/10.1111/j.1521-0391.2011.00186.x

Toronto Abolition Convergence. (2020). *An Indigenous abolitionist study guide.* Yellowhead Institute. https://yellowheadinstitute.org/2020/08/10/an-indigenous-abolitionist-study-group-guide/

Tucker, J. A., & Simpson, C. A. (2011). The recovery spectrum: From self-change to seeking treatment. *Alcohol Research & Health, 33*(4), 371-379. https://pubmed.ncbi.nlm.nih.gov/23580021

Venner, K. L., Donovan, D. M., Campbell, A. N. C., Wendt, D. C., Rieckmann, T., Radin, S. M., Momper, S. L., & Rosa, C. L. (2018). Future directions for medication assisted treatment for opioid use disorder with American Indian/Alaska Natives. *Addictive Behaviors, 86*, 111-117. https://doi.org/https://doi.org/10.1016/j.addbeh.2018.05.017

Venner, K. L., Greenfield, B. L., Vicuña, B., Muñoz, R., Bhatt, S., & O'Keefe, V. (2012). "I'm not one of them": Barriers to help-seeking among American Indians with alcohol dependence. *Cultural Diversity and Ethnic Minority Psychology, 18*(4), 352-362. https://doi.org/10.1037/a0029757

Ware, J. E., Kosinski, M., & Keller, S. D. (1996). A 12-item short-form health survey – Construction of scales and preliminary tests of reliability and validity. *Medical Care, 34*, 220-233. https://doi.org/10.1097/00005650-199603000-00003

Weng, H. Y., Fox, A. S., Shackman, A. J., Stodola, D. E., Caldwell, J. Z. K., Olson, M. C., Rogers, G. M., & Davidson, R. J. (2013). Compassion training alters altruism and neural responses to suffering. *Psychological science, 24*(7), 1171-1180. https://doi.org/10.1177/0956797612469537

Wenzel, S. L., Burnam, M. A., Koegel, P., Morton, S. C., Miu, A., Jinnett, K. J., & Sullivan, J. G. (2001). Access to inpatient or residential substance abuse treatment among homeless adults with alcohol or other drug use disorders. *Medical Care, 39*, 1158-1169. https://doi.org/10.1097/00005650-200111000-00003

White, W. L., & Miller, W. R. (2007). The use of confrontation in addiction treatment: History, science and time for change. *Counselor, 8*(4), 12-30.

White House, Executive Office of the President, & Office of National Drug Control Policy. (2022). *2022 National Drug Control Strategy.* https://www.whitehouse.gov/wp-content/uploads/2022/04/National-Drug-Control-2022Strategy.pdf

Winograd, R. P., Presnall, N., Stringfellow, E., Wood, C., Horn, P., Duello, A., Green, L., & Rudder, T. (2019). The case for a medication first approach to the treatment of opioid use disorder. *American Journal of Drug and Alcohol Abuse, 45*(4), 333-340. https://doi.org/10.1080/00952990.2019.1605372

Witkiewitz, K., Kranzler, H. R., Hallgren, K. A., Hasin, D. S., Aldridge, A. P., Zarkin, G. A., Mann, K. F., O'Malley, S. S., & Anton, R. F. (2021). Stability of drinking reductions and long-term functioning among patients with alcohol use disorder. *Journal of General Internal Medicine, 36*(2), 404-412. https://doi.org/10.1007/s11606-020-06331-x

Witkiewitz, K., Montes, K. S., Schwebel, F. J., & Tucker, J. A. (2020). What is recovery? *Alcohol Research: Current Reviews, 40*(3), 01-01. https://doi.org/10.35946/arcr.v40.3.01

Wurst, F. M., Skipper, G. E., & Weinmann, W. (2003). Ethyl glucuronide: The direct ethanol metabolite on the threshold from science to routine use. *Addiction, 98*(Suppl 2), 51–61. https://doi.org/10.1046/j.1359-6357.2003.00588.x

Zerger, S. (2002). *Substance abuse treatment: What works for homeless people? A review of the literature.* National Health Care for the Homeless Council.

9

Appendix: Tools and Resources

The following materials for your book can be downloaded free of charge once you register on the Hogrefe website:

Appendix 1: Safer-Use Strategies for Alcohol, Downers/Depressants, and Uppers/Stimulants
Appendix 2: Sample Letter for Mandated Treatment
Appendix 3: Short Inventory of Problems for Alcohol and Drugs – SIP-AD
Appendix 4: Progress Tracking Form
Appendix 5: Harm Reduction Goals Form
Appendix 6: SHaRE Form

How to proceed:

DOWNLOAD

1. Go to www.hgf.io/media and create a user account. If you already have one, please log in.

2. Go to **My supplementary materials** in your account dashboard and enter the code below. You will automatically be redirected to the download area, where you can access and download the supplementary materials.

   Code: B-PWGIAL

To make sure you have permanent direct access to all the materials, we recommend that you download them and save them on your computer.

Appendix 1: Safer-Use Strategies for Alcohol, Downers/Depressants, and Uppers/Stimulants

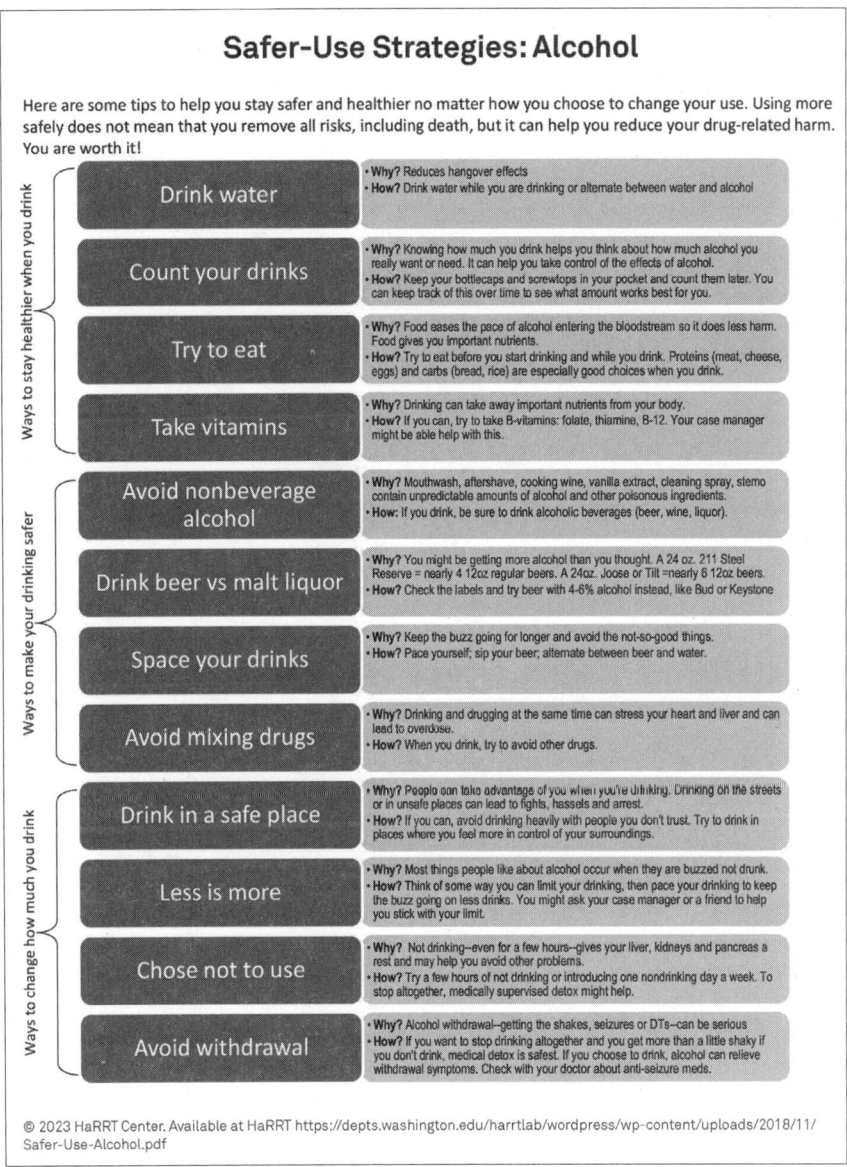

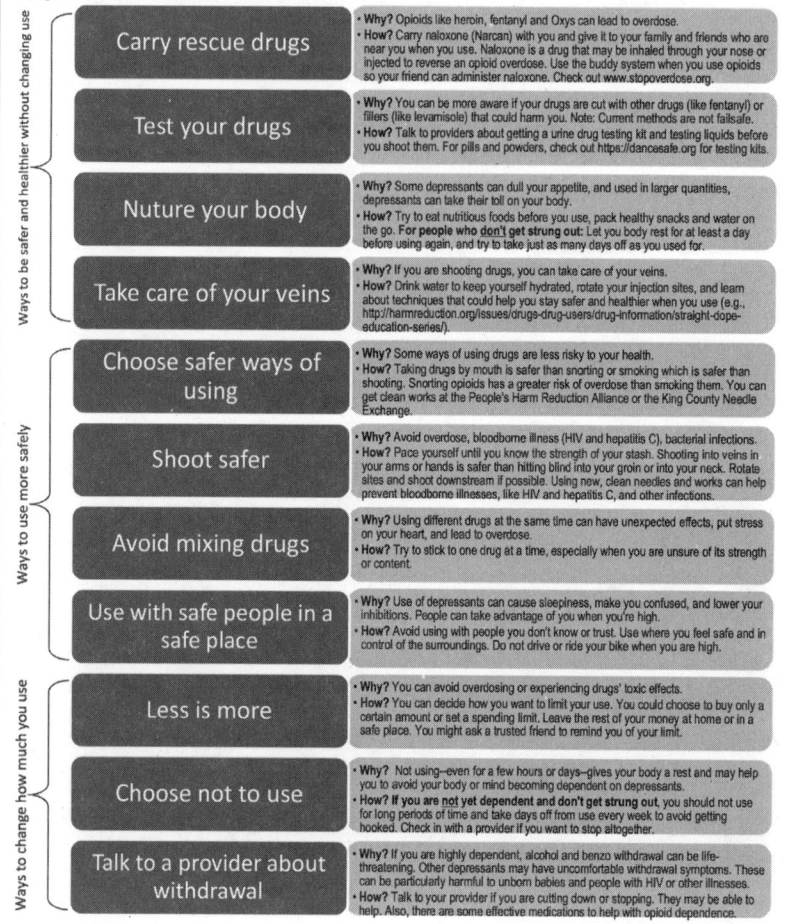

See p. 108 for instructions on how to obtain the full-sized, printable PDF.

9. Appendix: Tools and Resources

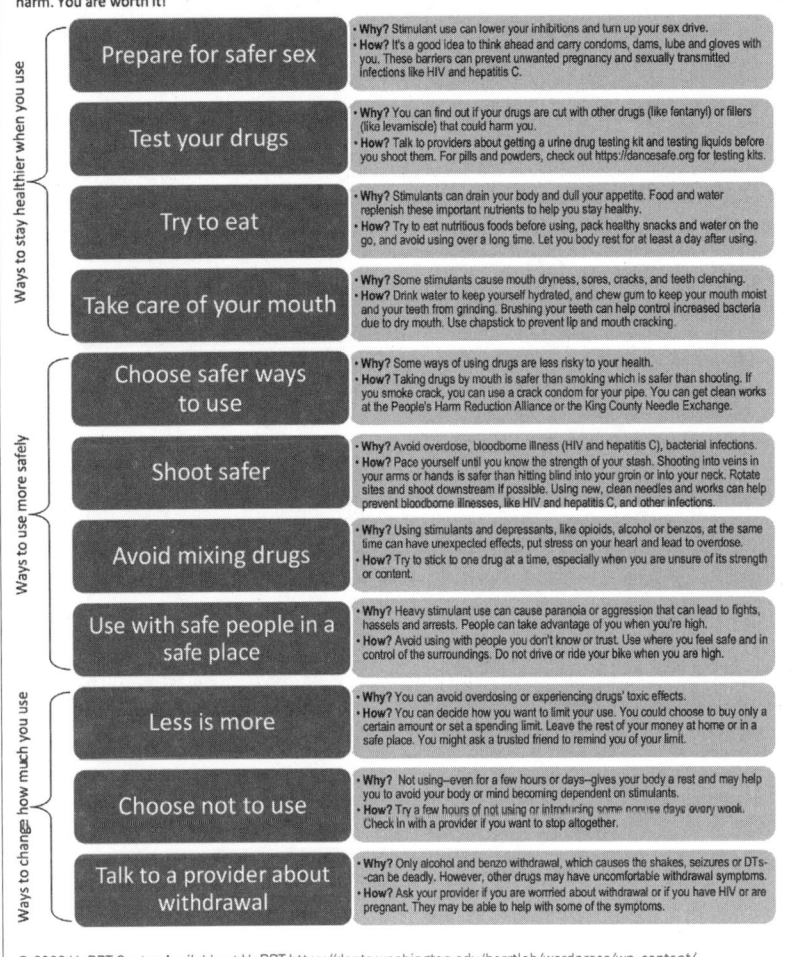

See p. 108 for instructions on how to obtain the full-sized, printable PDF.

Appendix 2: Sample Letter for Mandated Treatment

[Date]

RE: Confirmation of Harm Reduction Treatment Participation

Dear [entity that has mandated treatment]:

Per yours and my client's request, which is supported by [paperwork to ensure adherence to federal and state laws about disclosure of substance-use treatment information], *I am writing to confirm* [client name]'s *participation in an outpatient harm reduction treatment program through* [clinic name]. *Below, I describe this program and the client's participation as well as additional programming the client is currently attending.*

- **Harm reduction treatment at [clinic name]**. *On* [date], [client name] *sought out harm reduction treatment services with* [clinician name, license, position, NPI, etc]. *Harm reduction treatment entails a compassionate and pragmatic approach to help reduce substance-related harm and improve quality of life for people who use substances, and their communities, without requiring abstinence from substances or use reduction. It comprises three primary components delivered in weekly, 50-minute sessions. First, the client and clinician regularly assess and collaboratively track patterns of substance use and substance-related harm. Second, we establish and work toward harm reduction and quality-of-life goals. Third, we discuss ways to stay safer and healthier, even if a person is not able to stop using altogether.*
- *Since starting treatment on* [date], [client name] *has attended* [xx of xx] *weekly, scheduled appointments within the harm reduction treatment program at* [clinic name]. [If the client is interested and provides explicit approval, you may also describe treatment progress and milestones reached, as relevant.]

[As helpful and relevant, the client may wish you to name other programs and services in which the client is involved, as relevant, including psychiatry, supportive housing, primary care, mental health, case management, vocational training, mutual help, etc.]

Having this structure in place is important to [client name]'s *ongoing recovery, and they have established their commitment to it. Thank you for your support of this client and their recovery.*

Best regards,

See p. 108 for instructions on how to obtain the full-sized, printable PDF.

Appendix 3: Short Inventory of Problems for Alcohol and Drugs – SIP-AD

INSTRUCTIONS: I am going to read to you a number of events that people sometimes experience in relation to their alcohol/drug use. Please indicate how often each one has happened to you <u>during the past 30 days</u> by telling me the appropriate number (0 = never, 1 = once or a few times, etc.). If an item does not apply to you, answer zero (0).

	During the past 30 days, about how often has this happened to you?	Never (0)	Once or a few times (1)	Once or twice a week (2)	Daily or almost daily (3)
1.	I have been unhappy because of my drinking/drug use.				
2.	Because of my drinking/drug use, I have not eaten properly.				
3.	I have failed to do what is expected of me because of my drinking/drug use.				
4.	I have felt guilty or ashamed because of my drinking/drug use.				
5.	I have taken dangerous risks when I have been drinking/using drugs.				
6.	When drinking/using drugs, I have done impulsive things that I regretted later.				
7.	My physical health has been harmed by my drinking/drug use.				
8.	I have had money problems because of my drinking/drug use.				
9.	My physical appearance has been harmed by my drinking/drug use.				
10.	My family has been hurt by my drinking/drug use				
11.	A friendship or close relationship has been damaged by my drinking/drug use.				
12.	My drinking/drug use has gotten in the way of my growth as a person.				
13.	My drinking/drug use has damaged my social life, popularity, or reputation.				
14.	I have spent too much or lost a lot of money because of my drinking/drug use.				
15.	I have had an accident while drinking/using drugs/ intoxicated.				

Add columns: ____ + ____ + ____

Total: _____

Timeframe differs, but items based on W. R. Miller, J. S. Tonigan, & R. Longabaugh (1995), *The Drinker Inventory of Consequences (DrInC): An instrument for assessing adverse consequences of alcohol abuse. Test manual* (NIH Publication No. 95-3911). US Department of Health and Human Services, Public Health Service, National Institutes of Health, National Institute on Alcohol Abuse and Alcoholism. https://pubs.niaaa.nih.gov/publications/projectmatch/match04.pdf

See p. 108 for instructions on how to obtain the full-sized, printable PDF.

Appendix 4: Progress Tracking Form

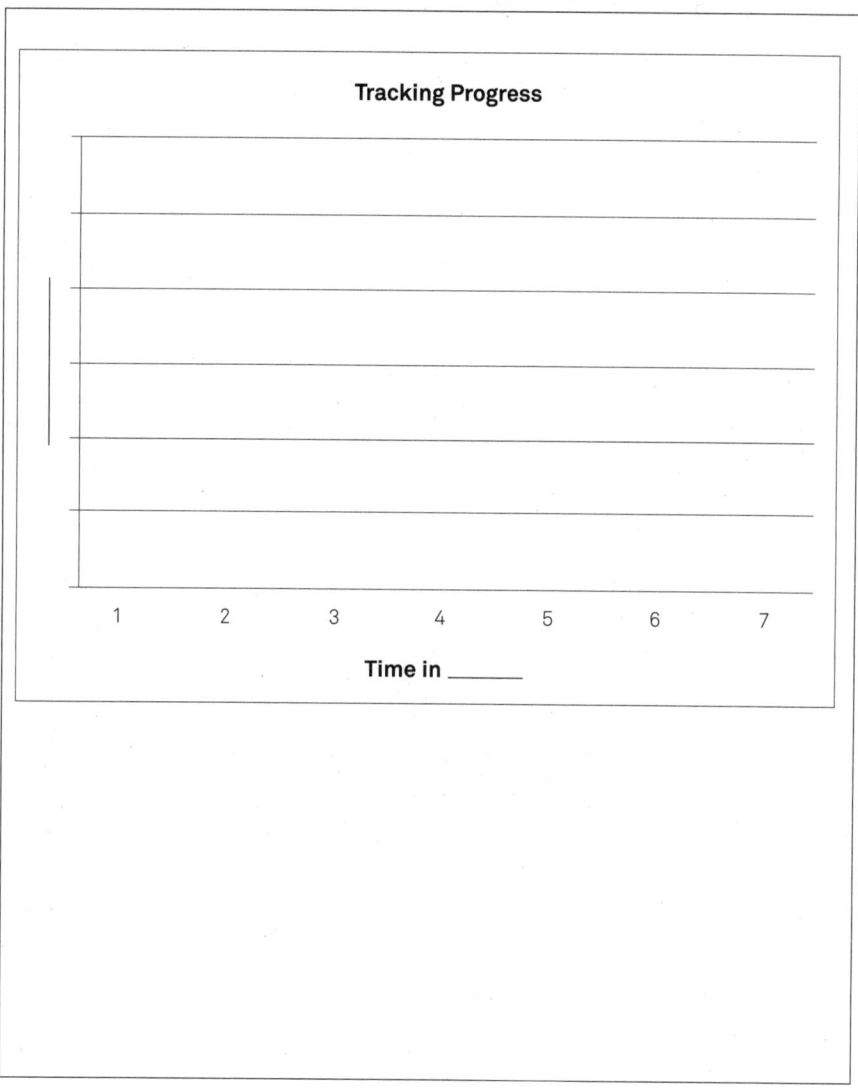

See p. 108 for instructions on how to obtain the full-sized, printable PDF.

Appendix 5: Harm Reduction Goals Form

What I want to make happen for myself

- _____
- _____
- _____
- _____
- _____
- _____
- _____
- _____

See p. 108 for instructions on how to obtain the full-sized, printable PDF.

Appendix 6: SHaRE Form

SHaRE Form		Week __ assessment of week __ goal	
Client's Stated Goals (week __)		Progress y/n	Achieved y/n
1			
2			
3			
4			
5			
6			
Week __ notes on progress towards goals since week __:			
		Week __ assessment of week __ plan	
Client's Safer-Use Plan (week __)		Achieved y/n	
1			
2			
3			
4			
5			
6			
Week __ notes on safer-use tips used since week __:			
Other notes/comments:			

See p. 108 for instructions on how to obtain the full-sized, printable PDF.

Advances in Psychotherapy
Evidence-Based Practice

Developed and edited with the support of the Society of Clinical Psychology (APA Division 12)

- Practice-oriented
- Evidence-based
- Expert authors
- Easy-to-read
- Compact
- Cost-effective

Editor-in-chief
Danny Wedding, PhD, MPH

Associate editors
Jonathan S. Comer, PhD
Linda Carter Sobell, PhD, ABPP
Kenneth E. Freedland, PhD
J. Kim Penberthy, PhD, ABPP

Latest releases

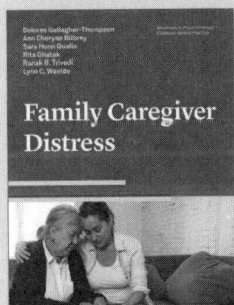

Family Caregiver Distress

Volume 50
ISBN 978-0-88937-517-8

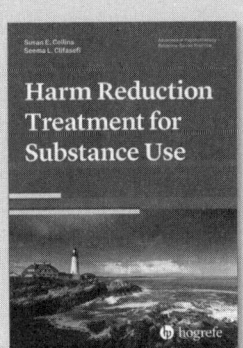

Harm Reduction Treatment for Substance Use

Volume 49
ISBN 978-0-88937-507-9

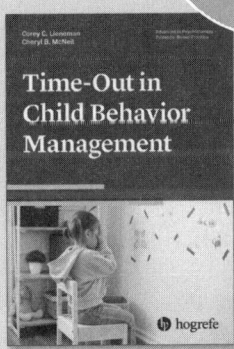

Time-Out in Child Behavior Management

Volume 48
ISBN 978-0-88937-509-3

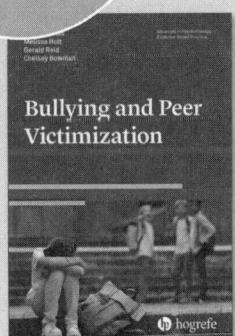

Bullying and Peer Victimization

Volume 47
ISBN 978-0-88937-408-9

www.hogrefe.com

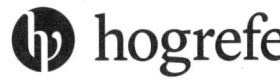

Advances in Psychotherapy
Evidence-Based Practice

Find out more at hgf.io/apt

All volumes of the series at a glance

Affirmative Counseling for Transgender and Gender Diverse Clients (Vol. 45)
Alcohol Use Disorders (Vol. 10)
Alzheimer's Disease and Dementia (Vol. 38)
ADHD in Adults (Vol. 35)
ADHD in Children and Adolescents (Vol. 33)
Autism Spectrum Disorder (Vol. 29)
Binge Drinking and Alcohol Misuse Among College Students and Young Adults (Vol. 32)
Bipolar Disorder (Vol. 1, 2nd ed.)
Body Dysmorphic Disorder (Vol. 44)
Childhood Maltreatment (Vol. 4, 2nd ed.)
Childhood Obesity (Vol. 39)
Chronic Illness in Children and Adolescents (Vol. 9)
Chronic Pain (Vol. 11)
Depression (Vol. 18)
Eating Disorders (Vol. 13)
Elimination Disorders in Children and Adolescents (Vol. 16)
Family Caregiver Distress (Vol. 50)
Generalized Anxiety Disorder (Vol. 24)
Growing Up with Domestic Violence (Vol. 23)
Harm Reduction Treatment for Substance Use (Vol. 49)
Headache (Vol. 30)
Heart Disease (Vol. 2)
Hoarding Disorder (Vol. 40)
Hypochondriasis and Health Anxiety (Vol. 19)
Insomnia (Vol. 42)
Internet Addiction (Vol. 41)
Language Disorders in Children and Adolescents (Vol. 28)
Mindfulness (Vol. 37)
Multiple Sclerosis (Vol. 36)
Nicotine and Tobacco Dependence (Vol. 21)
Nonsuicidal Self-Injury (Vol. 22)
Obsessive-Compulsive Disorder in Adults (Vol. 31)
Occupational Stress (Vol. 51)
Persistent Depressive Disorders (Vol. 43)
Phobic and Anxiety Disorders in Children and Adolescents (Vol. 27)
Problem and Pathological Gambling (Vol. 8)
Psychological Approaches to Cancer Care (Vol. 46)
Public Health Tools for Practicing Psychologists (Vol. 20)
Sexual Dysfunction in Women (Vol. 25)
Sexual Dysfunction in Men (Vol. 26)
Sexual Violence (Vol. 17)
Social Anxiety Disorder (Vol. 12)
Substance Use Problems (Vol. 15, 2nd ed.)
Suicidal Behavior (Vol. 14, 2nd ed.)
The Schizophrenia Spectrum (Vol. 5, 2nd ed.)
Time-Out in Child Behavior Management (Vol. 48)
Treating Victims of Mass Disaster and Terrorism (Vol. 6)
Women and Drinking: Preventing Alcohol-Exposed Pregnancies (Vol. 34)

Prices: US $29.80 / € 24.95 per volume. Standing order price US $24.80 / € 19.95 per volume (minimum 4 successive volumes) + postage & handling. Special rates for APA Division 12 and Division 42 members

www.hogrefe.com

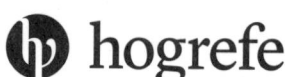